Almost Fifty Years' Experience as a Pediatrician

PAUL N. TSCHETTER, MD

Copyright © 2024 Paul N. Tschetter, MD
All rights reserved
First Edition

PAGE PUBLISHING
Conneaut Lake, PA

First originally published by Page Publishing 2024

ISBN 979-8-89157-010-8 (pbk)
ISBN 979-8-89157-020-7 (digital)

Printed in the United States of America

This book is dedicated to my wife, Renee, and my children, David, Jonathan, Stephen, Mark, Nicole, Michael, and Matthew. It is also dedicated to the many patients I was privileged to care for through the decades.

CONTENTS

Acknowledgments vii
Introduction ix
Chapter 1: Zachary and Tanner 1
Chapter 2: Medical Misadventures 11
Chapter 3: Death 30
Chapter 4: All Doctors Will Become Patients 38
Chapter 5: Dignity 50
Chapter 6: Short Stories 54
Chapter 7: Vaccines 88
Chapter 8: Mary Ann—A Grandfather's Perspective of a
 Tragedy 97
Epilogue 127

ACKNOWLEDGMENTS

To my son Mark N. Tschetter and Lynn Ozburn Davies,
for your time and help writing, researching,
proofing, and editing the manuscript.

INTRODUCTION

I saw my last patient on June 29, 2012, forty-nine years close to the day when I started practice on July 1, 1963. The fiftieth year was not to be. Shortly before noon, I closed all open windows on my computer because my computer access would be terminated at noon. My wife, Renee, and one of my sons finished clearing out my office. I gave my keys to the business manager and was told that the locks would be changed the next day.

I loved being a pediatrician, and I looked forward to work every day. Each day was a new adventure. My high school friends regularly reminded me that I had always wanted to be a doctor. During my internship, I cared for a baby with a heart defect called a coarctation of the aorta. I was fascinated by the case. Were all babies diagnosed with this condition born with it? Or could the condition develop after birth? Based on my interest in the case, I wrote an article about when the condition was diagnosed.

Dr. Henry Swan, Chief of Surgery at Colorado General Hospital, was so impressed with the article he offered me a residency in surgery. This was at the beginning of my junior year in medical school.

In the meantime, a new pediatrician in town, Dr. James Arthur, had me accompany him to the emergency room at Denver General Hospital. Dr. Arthur was always calm and engaged the parents in the evaluation of their sick child. Some cases were straightforward: infection, a sore throat, vomiting, and diarrhea. One case was not so clear. A five-month-old baby had a high fever and was breathing rapidly. When I listened to his chest, I heard no congestion. Dr. Arthur pointed out that the breath sounds on the left side were quite decreased. A chest X-ray showed a left-sided pneumonia. The Denver General Hospital emergency room experiences convinced me that I should be a pediatrician. Pediatricians care for children from birth to age twenty-one years and sometimes even older.

Over the years, many people have asked whether I regretted the choice to be a pediatrician. Up until 1985, pediatricians practiced medicine in a far different world than today. During the time I started practicing, there were no emergency room doctors, no neonatal nurse practitioners, no pagers, no cell phones, and no telephone services staffed by nurses to handle after-hours calls. As a pediatrician, if your patient went to the emergency room, you had to see them regardless of the hour, the weather, or any other circumstance. If there was an emergency C-section, you had to attend it whether night or day. You also had to handle all after-hours phone calls.

Throughout my career, I met countless pediatricians. A few of my early contemporaries quit after too many late-night telephone calls or too many middle-of-the-night trips to the emergency room. However, most pediatricians I met along the way worked hard and knew this was the life they had chosen.

For the first twenty years of my career, I practiced with one other pediatrician, Dr. Frits Mijer. We traded off being on call every other evening, all night, and every other weekend. Obviously, such a commitment took me away from my family at times. Missing the occasional family dinner and child activity is my only regret. Like nearly all parents, I love each of my seven children. I take great joy in the fact that they would tell you I rarely missed one of their activities, despite the significant intrusion into what most other folks would consider free time or family time.

The idea for this book came to me when I noticed there were medical treatments no longer being used today because they are ineffective or, even worse, they are harmful. I also wanted to share two very personal stories: my grandson's malignant brain tumor and the death of my granddaughter at age three days.

Before long I added several other topics and interesting cases including deaths, vaccines, etc. Woven into some of these memories are contributions made to the community by myself and others. Looking back to 1960, I have witnessed many major advances in medicine. In medical school, my biochemistry book (copyright

1953) had one sentence on deoxyribonucleic acid (DNA). The genetic code, DNA, plays an unbelievable role in medicine today. A monumental discovery by Crick and Watson in 1953 showed the structure of DNA as a double helix.

In one of his books, Dr. Lewis Thomas, MD, recounted that his father, a family practitioner in the early twentieth century, had only two effective drugs available. These were digitalis and morphine. At that time, life expectancy was just over forty years. Since then an additional thirty-plus years have been added.

During my almost-fifty-year medical career, I have witnessed many miraculous medical advances, including the development of many new drugs and vaccines. In 1960, the ability of a machine to examine the human body was limited to X-rays. Now computed tomography (CT) scans, ultrasounds, and magnetic resonance imaging (MRI) allow all parts of the body to be visualized and analyzed with amazing precision. Transplantation was just starting. Now hearts the size of walnuts are transplanted into very small infants. Liver and kidney transplantations are commonplace. Surgery advances include open-heart surgery, laparoscopic surgery, robotic surgery, and in utero fetal surgery, to name a few examples. Survival for some pediatric cancers has drastically improved. In 1963, the average survival rate for a child with acute lymphoblastic leukemia was six months. Today the cure rate is 85 percent to 90 percent.

Neonatology (premature baby or infant care) has made great strides. Ventilators for small premature babies and surfactant for immature lungs are among the advances that have greatly increased the survival rate for premature babies.

Early in the twenty-first century, the human genome project was completed. A new branch of medicine, medical genomics, was launched. Great strides were made in immunology and immunotherapy.

Over the years, I have read many fascinating books on medical advances. I particularly enjoyed *Emperors of all Maladies: A Biography of Cancer* and *The Gene: An Intimate History*, both written by the brilliant Siddhartha Mukherjee, MD. Another interesting book on the advancement of cancer treatments is *Cancerland: A Medical*

Memoir by David Scadden, MD. In the Great Courses (thegreatcourses.com), *What Science Knows About Cancer,* David Sadava, PhD (Adjunct Professor, City of Hope Medical Center, Claremont College), reports from the front line on the war against cancer.

For the families who entrusted their children to my care, I am extremely thankful. In the span of forty-nine years, I saw many second-generation families. When I left practice, I had five third-generation families.

Looking back, I would say the greatest joy has been the relationships I enjoyed with so many families.

My hope is that you will enjoy this book even if you are not a healthcare professional.

Paul N. Tschetter, MD
Greenwood Village, CO
2021

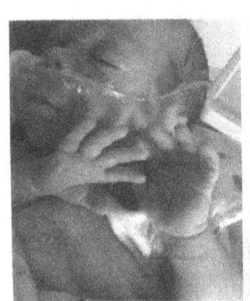

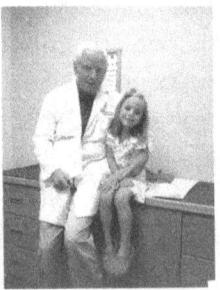

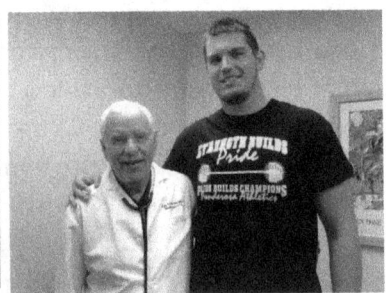

Pediatricians care for children from birth to 21 years old.
Pictured L to R: James, 1lb 14oz - Mae, 62 lbs - Sean 248 lbs

ALMOST FIFTY YEARS' EXPERIENCE AS A PEDIATRICIAN

Villager 8/16/12

Beloved Centennial pediatrician retires

Tschetter served community for nearly a half century

Dr. Nick Tschetter's last day of seeing patients at Pediatrics 5280 in Centennial was June 30 when he completed 49 years of caring for children in the southeast metro area.

"You have cared for me, my sisters and now my children for over 40 years," one parent recently said in a letter. Another wrote, "I was a first time mother. My husband just left me. Your kindness and reassuring manner was what I needed."

In addition to his work as a physician, Tschetter has been a dedicated community activist, especially as a longtime volunteer for Cherry Creek School District. He was physician for both the wrestling and football teams. When a child did not have money for a physical exam to participate in sports, Tschetter would see the child pro bono.

The veteran pediatrician was also active in the drug-policy and smoke-free committees and conducted work that ultimately led to a drug- and tobacco-free school district.

He received the Russell C. Polton Memorial award in 2004 for his service to CCSD.

In nominating Tschetter, Dr. James Shira noted Tschetter's leadership as a mentor to many young pediatricians. Coach Steve Foster said Tschetter always found time to listen and help.

Tschetter was very active in teaching at Children's Hospital and received the Career Teaching Scholar Award. He also served as medical staff president and on multiple hospital-related committees. He was awarded an Outstanding Service Award for his many contributions.

In 2007, Tschetter took the prestigious James E. Strain Award, which is given annually to a practitioner who exemplifies the ideals of the American Academy of Pediatrics.

Tschetter's partner, Dr. Julie Deckerman, called Tschetter an "exemplary pediatrician with an exemplary soul ... who can always be counted in the time of need to be a friend."

In 1997 after his 8-year-old grandson Zachary was diagnosed with a malignant brain tumor and underwent extensive treatments at Children's Hospital, Tschetter raised $1.5 million for the hospital. He also served on the board of Brent's Place, which provides housing for families whose children are undergoing cancer treatment at Children's Hospital.

Families have expresses sadness about Tschetter's departure from the practice.

"We had hoped to get both boys to 18 before you left," a parent wrote in a recent letter. "We will miss the implicit trust we had in you, your incredible medical knowledge and you experience."

Tschetter wrote the following to his families:

The journey has been wonderful,

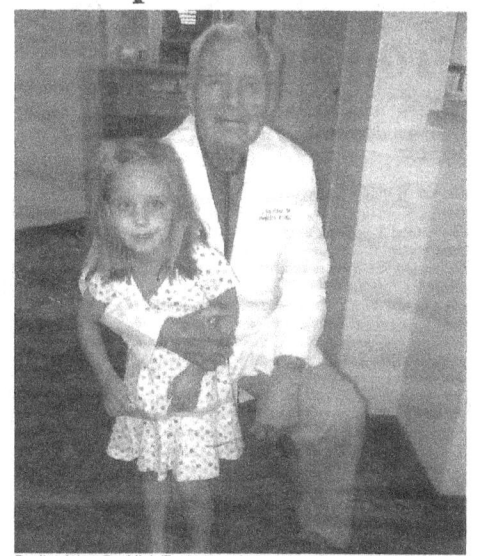

Pediatrician Dr. Nick Tschetter shares a moment with one of his many young patients, Mae McKenzie. Tschetter stopped practicing in June after nearly 50 years on the job at Centennial's Pediatrics 5280.
Photo courtesy of Nick Tschetter

and I thank each of you for the privilege of being a part of your lives.

For many of you, the relationship started with the birth of your child. For many others, you were my patient, and now I am caring for your child. And for a few, your child is actually the third generation for whom I have cared.

These long-term relationships are one of the true joys of being a pediatrician. Sharing in and helping with the joys and sorrows that are part of raising children has been a true honor for me.

This is your one and only chance to raise your children. Take good care of them. Show them your love daily. Your children are precious beyond words. May God bless your family in the days to come.

With affection and wishing you the best,

Dr. Tschetter

Villager Newspaper article featuring the author. Aug 16, 2012

xiii

COMMENTS AND OBSERVATIONS BY PARENTS AND PATIENTS

- To save money, some parents would ask me if the medicine was over the counter. Other parents would ask if the medicine was behind the counter or under the counter.
- "My son is having a problem with his temper mentality," one parent expressed.
- A five-year-old girl to her seven-year-old brother who was having a checkup, "My doctor has the same toys that your doctor has." (I was also the sister's doctor.)
- A mother told me her daughter was having a bad case of "gang green."
- I asked a mother if the baby had any trouble with his DPT immunization. His brother said, "I know what that spells! Poop!"

CHAPTER 1

Zachary and Tanner

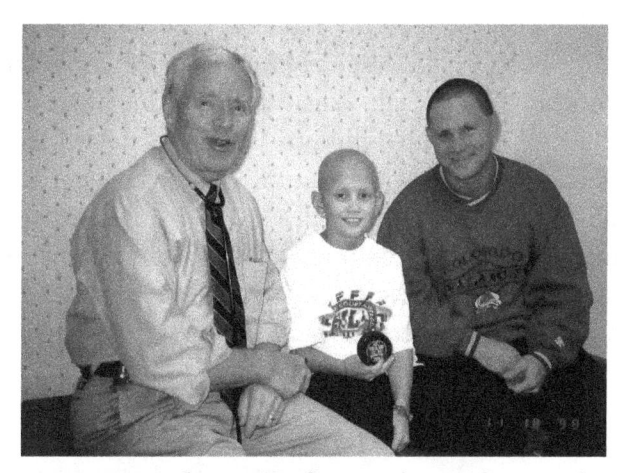

L-R: Dr. Tschetter (author) with grandson Zach Tschetter and son Stephen Tschetter

Zachary Tschetter

Christmas 1997. We were celebrating Christmas at our home in the mountains with all our children and grandchildren. My son Stephen said he needed some Tylenol for my grandson, Zach, as he was having a headache. In retrospect, Zach seemed somewhat subdued for the entire weekend. About ten days later when one of my partners saw Zach at the office for his headache, she thought it was probably just a virus. The following week his mother brought him in again as he had vomited once. One of my other partners stepped in and said Zach should have a CT scan. It was Tuesday, which was my day off. My partner who suggested the CT scan called me at home and said, "Your grandson has a brain tumor." It was felt that I should tell Zach's mother that he had a tumor. I immediately drove to my office to inform Zach's mother, Collette. This is every mother's worst nightmare.

Arrangements were made for the neuro-oncologists at Denver Children's Hospital to see Zach. Dr. Foreman was the first neuro-oncologist that had ever worked at Denver Children's Hospital. He had arrived from England just the year before. I had previously heard him give a talk, and he had remarked that of his first fifty-two pediatric patients with brain tumors, forty-nine had died.

Driving to Denver Children's Hospital my mind was racing and I had Zach dead and buried. When we arrived at the hospital, we were greeted by Dr. Garcia, who was head of oncology. He calmed me down and said that many brain tumors were now quite treatable.

An MRI was performed, which gave us a more detailed look at the tumor. The radiologist thought it might be an astrocytoma, which is not malignant. Zach was given Decadron to decrease the swelling of his brain. Surgery was scheduled for three days later.

When Zach was wheeled from the operating room to the recovery room, I asked him how his headache was. He smiled and said it was gone.

Many family members were in the waiting room anxiously waiting for Dr. Foreman to tell us what they had found. The tumor was a medulloblastoma, which is malignant. Dr. Foreman met with Zach's mother and father and myself. Dr. Foreman told us that if the tumor were to reoccur, the survival rate was…he drew a great big 0 on his yellow notepad.

The treatment protocol was designed by The Children's Hospital[*] oncology group. The treatment would follow one of two plans. All the children would have surgery and radiation. Then they all would receive two therapeutic drugs. Afterward, some children

---

[*] The Children's Hospital is now Children's Hospital Colorado.

would receive a third drug, let's call it A, and the other half would receive a different third drug, B. This is how new protocols are decided. If one group does better than the other group, then the third treatment will be the drug that worked best. Halfway through this study, it was determined that the group Zach was in was doing better than the other group. At that point, all the children received the same third drug.

The chemotherapy started immediately after the surgery. Three weeks after his surgery, Zach played in two roller hockey games. He wore a helmet. In the second game, he scored eight goals.

The chemotherapy was administered intravenously. This meant many trips to the hospital, and the therapy usually took one full day. During the therapy, Zach had one episode of fever. Children on chemotherapy have a marked decrease in their ability to fight infection. Any fever is treated by hospitalization, blood and spinal fluid cultures are taken, and intravenous antibiotics are administered. The cultures were all negative, and Zach went home after forty-eight hours of treatment.

Several weeks later, the radiation started. The radiation field included Zach's head, spinal cord, heart, lungs, and abdomen. The radiation made Zach violently ill with nausea and nonstop vomiting. My son Stephen, Zach's father, asked if Zach really needed to have the radiation. I stressed to him that the protocol must be followed exactly as it is written.

Well-meaning friends suggested various things such as vitamins might be helpful. Dr. Foreman was consulted, and he stressed that Zach should not receive any of these supplements. He said that some of the alternatives work by decreasing the activity of the therapeutic drugs.

During the therapies, Zach tried to go to school unless he was just feeling terrible. He lost all his hair and wore a baseball cap. A friend arranged a tour of the Air Force Academy, and we met Coach Fisher DeBerry. The coach started to hand Zach an Air Force visor. I shook my head, and Coach DeBerry immediately realized that a baseball cap would be better since Zach had no hair. Zach's father also shaved his head.

Therapy ended in about one year. After that, Zack had MRIs every three months for several years, then every six months, and finally once a year. He also had regular checkups in the oncology clinic.

After several years, Zach's life became more normal. He attended school and played baseball. I took him skiing, and he seemed to get very tired. He kept up all day. It was sometime later that I realized that we were at 11,000 feet and Zach had a hemoglobin of 8 grams per deciliter. (A normal pediatric hemoglobin is roughly 10.9–14.5 grams per deciliter.)

Zach is considered cured of his brain tumor. He completed high school and played varsity baseball for three years. Zach is now thirty-four years old, and twenty-nine years have passed since the diagnosis of a brain tumor. He works, and he loves to snowboard. He counts every day as a blessing.

ALMOST FIFTY YEARS' EXPERIENCE AS A PEDIATRICIAN

Tanner Seebaum

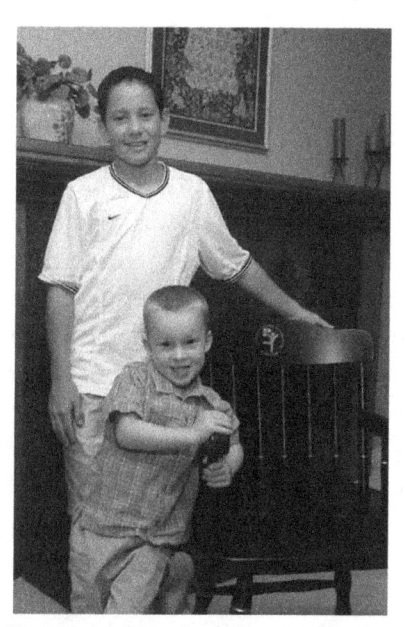

***Tanner Seebaum (front) and Zach Tschetter (back) with the Children's Hospital Colorado Neuro-Oncology Chair*`

Tanner became a patient of mine sometime after his second birthday. He was referred to my practice by Dr. Nick Foreman. Dr. Foreman was the same general oncologist who had treated my grandson Zach. Dr. Foreman felt that since I had experience with the treatment of my grandson, I would be a good fit to care for Tanner. Tanner was born in Texas, and around eighteen months of age his parents noticed that he was regressing with milestones. He often cried while repeating "my head, my head" along with some vomiting. At the time, he was taken to his pediatrician in Texas, who felt that he just had ear infections.

The Seebaums moved to the Denver area in the summer of 1998 when Tanner was twenty-two months old. Shortly after their move, Tanner's condition worsened. Being new to the area, the Seebaums did not have a pediatrician yet. Tanner's grandmother was a pediatric nurse in Cheyenne, Wyoming. She also noticed Tanner's poor health and said that Tanner needed to go to Cheyenne to be seen at the clinic where she worked. He was seen by a pediatrician in Cheyenne, the same pediatrician Tanner's mother saw as a child. Upon his visit to the pediatrician in Cheyenne, a CT scan was ordered, and it was discovered that Tanner had a brain tumor. Tanner was immediately referred to Children's Hospital in Denver. The Seebaums returned to Denver, and Tanner was admitted to Children's Hospital Denver.

After initial surgery, Tanner was diagnosed with a malignant ependymoma at the age of twenty-two months. Dr. Michael Handler, a pediatric neurosurgeon, performed his surgery. This is the same neurosurgeon that had completed Zach's surgery. Tanner then received chemotherapy for a number of months. Because of his young age, he did not receive any radiation as it is extremely devastating to the brain of young children.

The location of the tumor was such that it blocked the flow of Tanner's cerebral spinal fluid. He had to have a shunt that drained the spinal fluid into his abdomen. On a number of occasions, this shunt became blocked, and he had to have a revision of the shunt. Once the blockage was corrected, his symptoms immediately went away. After one of the revisions, he seemed disheartened. When asked what he needed to make him feel better, he said he wanted crackers and 7Up. After several bites of cracker and several sips of the 7Up, he broke out into a smile. Life was good again.

Over the years, Tanner had several recurrences of his tumor. He required surgery again in 2001 and 2004. Each surgery was followed by six weeks of radiation as there seemed to be no other options. Tanner enjoyed eight years of remission. He was quite healthy, attended school, performed well in his academics, and participated in the normal activities of a young child.

In May of 2012, his brain tumor recurred yet again. This time, it was not only the ependymoma but also a glioblastoma. Surgery was not possible as he had many, many tumors. There was no effective treatment. Tanner and his family were informed that he had only months to live.

Undaunted, Tanner continued to live the last year of his life to the fullest. He started by getting his driver's permit and learned to drive. Next he repelled off a forty-story skyscraper. He vacationed at many places he loved. He continued to work out daily. Since he loved music and technology, he decided to become a disc jockey (DJ). This became a passion, and he was soon recognized as a real talent. He regularly received invitations to DJ at many venues in the Denver area. The DJ community in Denver put together an amazing benefit for Tanner. DJs from far and wide flew to Denver to play for free. Despite worsening symptoms, Tanner opened for the headliner, and he brought down the house.

Tanner's finale topped them all. He was invited to DJ at the Hard Rock Cafe in Denver, and he was barely able to get out of his wheelchair. Then amazing strength came back to him as he began to perform. Tanner's final gig was the Beatport Live, an international event that attracts DJs from around the world.

Sadly, Tanner lost his battle with cancer on July 12, 2013, just before his seventeenth birthday. Tanner inspired many people in the way he lived his life. His career in music affected many of his friends as well as many people he had never met.

PAUL N. TSCHETTER, MD

TCH NEWS — JUNE 2002 — The Children's Hospital — Denver, Colorado — www.TheChildrensHospital.org

Grateful grandparents endow a chair in Neuro-Oncology

By Wendy S. Meyer, Foundation

Two families have come together to establish The Tanner Seebaum and Zachary Tschetter Chair in Neuro-Oncology through gifts totaling $1.6 million. Grateful grandparents of two young boys who were treated at Children's led the efforts to fund the chair with the help of their families and friends. Nicholas Foreman, MD, director of Neuro-Oncology and associate professor of Pediatrics and Neurosurgery at the University of Colorado Health Sciences Center, will hold this esteemed position.

Carol McMurry, grandmother of Tanner Seebaum, and Nick Tschetter, MD, grandfather of Zach Tschetter, spearheaded the effort. "Every day we are so thankful for the time we have with our grandsons that we wanted to do something to honor them. At the same time, we wanted to support Dr. Foreman and the Neuro-Oncology program because of the outstanding clinical and research work they do," McMurry said.

According to Dr. Tschetter, "Keeping the department of Neuro-Oncology strong and making it even stronger offers the most hope to Zach and the many children who depend on The Children's Hospital for care."

As a community pediatrician for more than 38 years and former president of the medical board at the hospital, Dr. Tschetter has strong ties to Children's. Four years ago, his grandson was diagnosed with a brain tumor. At that point, Dr. Tschetter's relationship with Children's drastically changed as he became a family member of a patient rather than a doctor. "Zach received not only the best technical, cutting-edge medicine there is, but the physicians who gave that care did it with dignity and utmost concern for Zach and his family," Tschetter said.

A former medical librarian, McMurry became involved with Children's when her grandson Tanner was diagnosed with a brain tumor at 21 months. Today Tanner is 5 years old and Zach is 11. Dr. Foreman and his team treated both boys.

Support from the chair will allow Children's to establish a training program to educate future neuro-oncologists; expand vital research to improve therapies; and provide an important measure of financial stability for Neuro-Oncology. Since establishing the program in 1994, Dr. Foreman has developed a comprehensive, multidisciplinary program that has served 272 children from the Rocky Mountain region and across the country. Children's is extremely fortunate to have Dr. Foreman, as there are only 60 pediatric neuro-oncologists in the world.

"The chair enables the Neuro-Oncology program to grow further – from one of the best in the world, to the best and most innovative. It will be as strong in research as in clinical care," Dr. Foreman said.

See GRATEFUL on Page 2

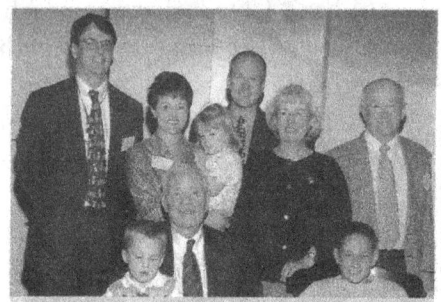

Family and friends of Dr. Nick Tschetter and Carol McMurry celebrate a new endowed chair for Children's. From left to right are: Dr. Nick Foreman, chairholder, Stephanie Seebaum, Ellie Seebaum, Matt Seebaum, Carol McMurry and Pat Spieles. Seated: Tanner Seebaum, Dr. Nick Tschetter and Zach Tschetter.

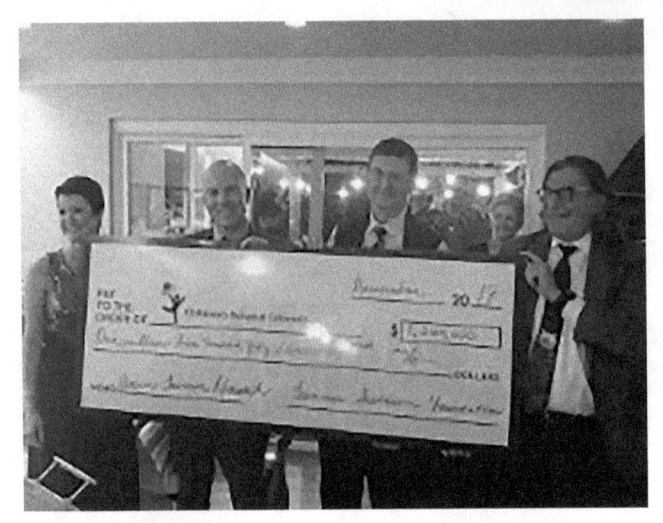

The Seebaums presenting a check to Children's Hospital Colorado Neurology

ALMOST FIFTY YEARS' EXPERIENCE AS A PEDIATRICIAN

Tanner Seebaum and Zachery Tschetter Chair
Pediatric Neuro-Oncology

The journeys of these young men were recognized by the Tanner Seebaum and Zachary Tschetter Chair in Pediatric Neuro-Oncology at Denver Children's Hospital. To show our gratitude for the care Tanner and Zach received, the families agreed to launch a campaign to raise $1.5 million to endow this Chair in Neuro-Oncology. I spearheaded the project. Tanner's paternal grandmother, Carol McMurry, was a major contributor. The McMurry and Seebaum families have since contributed funds for several other endowed chairs.

Tanner Seebaum Foundation

Tanner's parents, Matt and Stephanie, started a foundation in Tanner's name to raise money for research in pediatric brain tumors. They closed the foundation in 2019 after raising over $1.3 million.

Brent's Place

Brent's Place is a facility of *safe-clean* apartments that houses families whose children are getting bone marrow transplants. Donn and Linda Eley started Brent's Place in memory of their son, Brent, who died after an unsuccessful bone marrow transplant. One of the units is called Tanner's House. Tanner's paternal grandmother, Carol McMurry, was the major donor.

COMMENTS AND OBSERVATIONS BY PATIENTS AND PARENTS

- A little four-year-old boy watched the receptionist feed the fish. She explained to him that the fish get shrimp once daily and the next day they get dry fish food. The little boy then asked, "Do they ever get water?"
- A five-year-old boy watched me write a prescription. He asked if it was in cursive. I said yes, it was cursive. He then said, "My brother can talk cursive."
- I was performing a throat culture on a six-year-old. I asked her if she could say a big ah. She then said, "Big ah."
- The nurse warned me that my next patient, a four-year-old boy, had a question for me. I walked into the room, and he looked at me and asked, "Are you a professional?"
- A seven-year-old told me I should not be seeing sick patients as it was a Sunday. He seemed satisfied when I told him that Jesus healed on Sundays.

CHAPTER 2

Medical Misadventures

Over the course of my career, pediatric medicine has significantly evolved. Many standard practices and procedures changed, or became obsolete, because they were ineffective or, even worse, they were detrimental to the child's health.

Clysis

Premature newborn fluid requirements are calculated daily. If a premature infant's fluid was insufficient and could not be met orally, additional fluids were given by clysis. During the clysis procedure, a long needle was placed in the subcutaneous tissue along the side of the infant's spine. Fluid was injected as the needle was slowly removed. The invention of the butterfly needle made clysis obsolete. Before the butterfly needle infusion was invented, it was very difficult to give intravenous (IV) fluids to very small babies.

pHisoHex (hexachlorophene)

Shortly after birth, babies were bathed with this antibacterial detergent. Infants demonstrating irritability, convulsions, and cerebral rigidity were linked to pHisoHex. It was found to be a neurotoxin. During autopsies, infant brains were examined and vacuolization of cells was noted. Vacuolization causes irreversible brain injury.

Accordingly, around 1970, the bathing of newborns with pHisoHex was discontinued.

Sleep position

For years, babies slept in the position their parents thought was most comfortable for the infant. In 1990, a New Zealand study showed a 60 percent decrease in sudden infant death syndrome (SIDS) when babies slept on their backs. In the United States, most pediatricians now recommend that infants be placed on their backs for sleep.

Pyralgin

This drug was a very effective antipyretic. Antipyretics reduce fevers and keep them down. In 1970, a very serious effect on bone marrow associated with the use of Pyralgin was noted. It was found that Pyralgin greatly decreased the production of white blood cells. Perhaps more important, when using Pyralgin, both physicians and parents were lulled into thinking the child's infection was getting better. Masking symptoms can be very dangerous and misleading. Pyralgin is no longer used.

Transporting premature and sick infants

In the past, doctors themselves transported fragile, premature, and sick babies to Denver Children's Hospital. The premature babies were placed in a small aluminum box with a glass window to observe the baby. To keep the baby warm, a hot water bottle was placed in the box. A bottle of oxygen was also strapped to the box with the end of the tubing placed next to the infant's nose. At the time, ventilators for infants did not exist.

In 1965, L. Joseph Butterfield, MD, became the director of the Newborn Center at Denver Children's Hospital. Butterfield's goal was to regionalize newborn care. Over time, transportation was supplied by ambulance, helicopter, and airplane. Premature and sick infants were brought to Denver Children's Hospital's Newborn Center, and the infant mortality rate in Colorado dropped dramatically.

Streptococcal disease

During World War II, many streptococcal studies were done at the Warren Air Force Base in Wyoming. As a result, Wyoming was known as the strep capital of the United States. To eliminate strep throat in schools, all students were cultured weekly. Positive cases were treated. Soon there was very little strep in Wyoming schools. As a result, Wyoming children grew up with little contact with streptococcal disease and thus did not develop antibodies against strep. This later created an adult population that was as susceptible to strep as were children.

When I first went into practice, if a child had a positive throat culture for strep, the entire family was cultured. This was to find strep carriers who were infecting other members of the family. (One develops antibodies against strep by having the disease or being a carrier.) Even dogs were cultured to see if they were a carrier. Sometimes they were. Dogs were not allowed in the office, so I would go out to the parking lot to culture the dog and would hope the dog wasn't too aggressive.

The primary reason for treating strep throat was for the prevention of acute rheumatic fever and acute glomerulonephritis (a group of diseases that injure the kidneys). In the 1970s and into the early 1980s, there was very little acute rheumatic fever in the United States. As a result, infectious disease experts considered recommending ceasing the treatment of strep throat. Then in approximately 1985, an outbreak of acute rheumatic fever occurred in Utah. Salt Lake City had 136 pediatric cases. To resolve this outbreak, doctors continued to treat strep throat with antibiotics. Current practice today dictates cultures or a rapid strep test and treatment with antibiotics if results are positive. Other family members and the family dog are no longer cultured. If you are a strep carrier (no symptoms), your body is making antibodies against strep, and this is good.

Chickenpox and German measles infection parties

At one time it was recommended that exposing children to these two illnesses was a good idea. Parents would literally host a party for the neighborhood kids to expose them. Cake, ice cream, and chickenpox! The thinking behind these parties was that both viruses were believed to be mild illnesses and one might as well get it over with. This practice is no longer recommended. Every year there are about two hundred deaths from chickenpox. Most of the deaths from chickenpox are caused by secondary infections, such as flesh-eating strep.

Exposing children to German measles (rubella) carries significant risks if the child's mother is pregnant. The exposed child can pass the virus to their mother, and if the mother is in the late first trimester of pregnancy, the fetus can be badly damaged. Potential damage to the fetus includes heart defects, visual problems, and mental retardation. We now have effective vaccines against both chickenpox and German measles.

Thalidomide

Thalidomide was introduced as a cancer drug in West Germany in 1957. However, many doctors used it off-label to treat sleep problems and morning sickness. As a result, in the early 1960s, many children were born with phocomelia (shortened or absent limbs). Worldwide over 10,000 babies were affected. About 40 percent died shortly after birth. In 1962, the FDA declined to approve Thalidomide for use in the United States.

Perceived orthopedic problem

In the early 1960s, doctors started to realize that apparently abnormal indicators were part of normal child development. Babies are normally born with flat feet and bowed legs. Further, tibial torsion also results in babies' feet either toeing in or toeing out. Additionally, most children become knock-kneed at some point. These conditions were often treated with shoes (Thomas Heel) and splints (Denis Browne, a.k.a. Dennis-Brown). However, eventually doctors realized that these conditions were false indicators. Frequently doing nothing had the same results as the treatment. Most children's legs and feet straighten out and align eventually, and therefore these conditions are self-correcting. Tibial torsion and knock-knees are good examples of the importance of knowing medical history, because history will often indicate that no treatment or therapy is necessary.

Osgood-Schlatter disease

Osgood-Schlatter is a condition seen in adolescent children, especially those who are very active and involved in sports. There is pain and tenderness over the tibial tuberosity. The tibial tuberosity is the area where the tendon from the kneecap attaches to the tibia. Initially, treatment partially consisted of ice, rest, and analgesics (aspirin, acetaminophen, etc.). Occasionally, the leg was placed in a cylinder cast to rest the leg. When the condition was better understood, stretching and muscle building were added. Stretching the quadriceps, and especially the hamstrings, has greatly shortened the time of rehabilitation and expedited recovery. Treating by casting is now rare.

Scoliosis screening

Idiopathic adolescent scoliosis is the sideways curve of the spine (backbone). The cause is unknown. When I started practicing in 1963, schools often screened for scoliosis. This screening was done by a school nurse or a volunteer. The screening was not accurate, and many children were referred to their physician only to discover the child did not have scoliosis. Unfortunately, in the meantime, parents and children experienced high anxiety. Children made an unnecessary trip to the doctor and often had an X-ray and possible unnecessary treatment, e.g., a back brace.

In 2018, the Journal of the American Medical Association (JAMA) and the US Preventative Task Force felt there was insufficient evidence to make a recommendation for or against screening. In the Denver area, no school screening is conducted. Adolescents with signs and symptoms of back problems should see their pediatrician to diagnose back pain and/or noticeable curvature of the spine.

Acne

In the past, treatment for acne included eliminating French fries, hamburgers, cola drinks, and chocolate. All greasy foods were avoided even though diet seemed to make no difference. As the pathogenesis of acne became better understood, many good medications were developed. These medications included topical ointments to unblock hair follicles, topical and oral antibiotics to fight infection, etc. For severe scarring-type acne, an oral drug called Accutane was highly effective.

Hemolytic disease of the newborn (erythroblastosis fetalis)

This condition is caused when small amounts of the baby's blood cells get into the mother's circulation. The mother then makes antibodies against the baby's red blood cells, and these antibodies pass through the placenta to the baby, destroying the baby's red blood cells. This happens when the mother and baby have different blood types. For example, if the mother is Rh-negative and the baby is Rh-positive. This also occurs if the mother is type O and the baby is type A, B, or AB (collectively ABO). One of the breakdown products of red blood cells is called bilirubin, which is very toxic to a baby's brain. Elevated bilirubin makes the baby's skin yellow and is called jaundice. In addition, the baby becomes very anemic due to the breakdown of red blood cells. The liver processes bilirubin, but newborn babies have immature livers and therefore difficulty in processing bilirubin.

The Rh incompatibility is more serious than the ABO incompatibility. Prior to 1945, there was no treatment for Rh incompatibility, and about ten thousand babies died per year. The mortality rate from hemolytic disease for newborns during this time was approximately 50 percent. Thankfully, a procedure called exchange transfusion was introduced. The procedure was very effective but not without risk.

The next major breakthrough came in 1968 when the drug RhoGAM was developed. RhoGAM prevents the mother from producing antibodies after exposure to the baby's Rh-positive blood.

When fetal blood cells escape into the mother's circulation, RhoGAM binds them, making them invisible to the mother's immune system. RhoGAM has essentially eliminated hemolytic disease of newborns caused by the Rh factor.

Chloramphenicol (chloromycetin)

In 1947, the medical community hailed the discovery of the broad-spectrum antibiotic chloramphenicol, which was derived from a bacterium. However, two serious side effects were noted: One side effect was that it could cause aplastic anemia, which could be fatal. The second side effect was that it could cause gray baby syndrome in newborns. Gray baby syndrome is characterized by cardiovascular collapse and, if untreated, could lead to death. Because of these side effects, chloramphenicol is now rarely used in the United States. When it is used, it is sometimes used to treat typhoid fever because some strains of salmonella are resistant to more conventional therapies. Despite its potentially fatal side effects, and scant use in the United States, chloramphenicol is sold over the counter in some countries.

Tetracyclines

These broad-spectrum antibiotics were patented in 1953. Many years later it was noted that this class of drugs stains the permanent teeth of children. This staining was permanent and made worse by light. The front teeth were stained the most. After this staining was noted, tetracycline was not prescribed for children under the age of nine years unless it was absolutely necessary.

Diethylstilbestrol (DES)

DES is a synthetic estrogen (female hormone). DES was frequently prescribed by physicians from 1938 to 1971 to women who had previous miscarriages or premature births. DES had few known side effects for the women who took it, other than a small increased risk of breast cancer. Unfortunately, the offspring of mothers who were prescribed DES had significant problems. Daughters who were exposed to DES have an increased risk (forty times) of vaginal and cervical cancer. Sons exposed to DES have an increased risk of testicular cysts that are not cancerous. In 1971, the FDA advised doctors to stop using DES. It has yet to be determined whether the grandchildren of women who took DES are affected.

Ashtrays in the waiting room

Given today's smoking restrictions, it is almost unfathomable that pediatricians had ashtrays in their waiting rooms prior to 1964. The smoke undoubtedly was harmful to newborns and children with asthma, pneumonia, bronchiolitis, etc. In the mid-1960s, the surgeon general's report linking cigarettes to lung cancer was published. Ashtrays in the waiting room were immediately removed. There were few complaints.

House calls

When I first started practicing, doctors still made house calls. Families loved house calls, especially on a cold, snowy day. A physician could learn a lot by visiting a patient's home. Our house call fee was ten dollars versus five dollars for an office visit. House calls were not eliminated because they were expensive; they were eliminated because of logistical and other considerations (time, distance from the office, no lab or X-ray, no nurse support, etc.).

ALMOST FIFTY YEARS' EXPERIENCE AS A PEDIATRICIAN

Hyaline membrane disease of the newborn (respiratory distress syndrome, or RDS)

This breathing difficulty is very common in premature infants. Respiratory distress syndrome (RDS) occurs in 50 percent of premature babies born between twenty-four and thirty weeks. RDS is caused by a deficiency of surfactant in the lungs. Before ventilators were developed for infants, many RDS babies would die. All RDS babies that could not breath on their own would die. RDS babies also become very acidotic (acidic blood). To treat acidosis, neonatologist Robert H. Usher, MD, recommended giving intravenous sodium bicarbonate to these infants depending how acidotic they were. Over time (fifty years), it became evident that not only was this treatment ineffective but was very harmful. The Usher regiment affected cerebral blood flow, causing intracranial hemorrhaging, decreased oxygen delivery to tissues, and affected cardiac function. In 1980, the medical community had developed surfactant replacement therapy, greatly benefiting premature babies with RDS.

Smallpox (Variola)

Smallpox was a devastating viral illness. The mortality rate was over 30 percent. In the twentieth century alone, the number of deaths worldwide caused by smallpox was estimated to have been between three hundred and five hundred million. Smallpox started with fever and was followed by fluid-filled sores that turned into a pox with a dent in the center. Around 1800, Edward Jenner introduced a smallpox vaccine. He used the cowpox virus. In the twentieth century, the World Health Organization (WHO) began a campaign to eliminate smallpox. The last case of smallpox in the United States was in 1952.

In the early 1960s, C. Henry Kempe, MD, at the University of Colorado Department of Pediatrics, strongly recommended that smallpox vaccination should be discontinued in the United States.

Dr. Kempe rightfully argued that vaccinating was causing more deaths than it was preventing. The last reported death from smallpox occurred in 1978. The WHO reported the global eradication of smallpox in 1980.

PAUL N. TSCHETTER, MD

Rectal suppositories to stop vomiting

Suppositories such as Phenergan and Compazine were widely used to stop vomiting. However, they may mask symptoms of very serious conditions. These include illnesses such as meningitis, pneumonia, and bowel obstruction (such as intussusception midgut volvulus). We learned that it was better to rest the intestinal tract. After a period, if there was no further vomiting, small amounts of electrolyte solution (Pedialyte) was given to prevent dehydration. Persistent vomiting requires medical evaluation.

Bendectin

This combination of two drugs, plus vitamin B6, was introduced in the 1950s. The drug was very effective in treating nausea and vomiting during pregnancy (morning sickness). Over thirty million pregnant women were treated with this medication worldwide. In the 1970s, Bendectin lawsuits alleged the drug caused birth defects. Over a thousand lawsuits were filed, and these lawsuits received wide publicity. Merrell Dow Pharmaceuticals refused to settle any Bendectin litigation. They won thirty-seven of thirty-nine cases that ultimately were brought to trial. According to the Journal of the American Medical Association (JAMA), the Federal Drug Administration (FDA) never concluded Bendectin caused birth defects. Merrell Dow ceased production of the drug in 1983 because the cost of defending the lawsuits was greater than the company's profits. Bendectin is an example of how litigation can impact drugs and medical procedures. Even though the studies were inconclusive, the lawsuits ultimately sank it.

Tonsillectomy and Adenoidectomy (T&A)

Tonsillectomy & Adenoidectomy (T&A) is one of the most common surgical procedures done in the world. In the United States, it is the third most common procedure. Many believe that President

Washington died of a peritonsillar abscess (an infection around the tonsil).

From the 1950s to 1970s, 1,400,000 T&As were conducted annually. A study in 1934 showed that 61 percent of New York school children had a tonsillectomy. The current rate is about 200,000 per year.

T&As are not without risk. Children may die from the anesthetic or hemorrhage. The current death rate is 1 per 15,000 operations. When the United States was doing 1.4 million T&As per year, this translated into about 100 deaths annually.

In years past, T&As were performed for all sorts of problems. One of the indications for a T&A is sleep apnea. Another indication is for chronic otitis media with effusion.

When I was a child, having a T&A was a rite of passage. However, my two sisters and I did not have this procedure because my parents had no insurance and did not have the money to pay out of pocket. The procedure was so successful and popular because it was performed when a child was about 5 or 6 years old. The doctor could almost guarantee that a child would have fewer upper respiratory illnesses after a T&A. Ironically, even children who did not have the procedure also had less illness. You see, after the ages of 5 to 6 years, every child develops additional immunity from having illnesses, including respiratory illnesses.

How T&As affect the immune system is controversial. Studies have shown a wide range of illnesses that seemed more prevalent after a T&A. Because the benefits of T&As have never been conclusively established, today's practitioners only recommend this procedure when a definite medical condition will be improved by removing the tonsils and adenoids. The most common indication is sleep apnea that can be due to enlarged tonsils and adenoids. At one time, pediatricians performed tonsillectomies, but rarely if ever perform them now. Most of these surgeries are performed by an otolaryngologist. The huge reduction of tonsillectomies has greatly decreased the number of routine surgeries performed on children.

Thymus gland radiation

The thymus gland is situated on either side of the upper trachea (windpipe). At one time, its function was unknown. Eventually, it was learned that the thymus gland produces the hormone Thymosin. Thymosin stimulates the production of disease fighting T-cells (white blood cells). T-cells play an important role protecting the body against autoimmune diseases (diseases where the immune system turns against itself).

On some chest X-rays, the thymus was noted to be very large. The concern with a large thymus was that it could block the airway. Because it shrunk the gland, radiation was used to treat some children with large thymuses. By today's standards, the amount of radiation used was high. Because the radiation caused many cases of thyroid cancer years after it was administered, the practice of shrinking the thymus with radiation was discontinued in the early 1960s. The cancer resulting from efforts to shrink the thymus with radiation was a tragic and unnecessary result because the thymus shrinks and is gone by puberty.

Urinary tract infections (UTIs)

After a child's first UTI, the evaluation protocol became quite aggressive with part of the evaluation requiring a general anesthetic. The first step in evaluating a UTI was an intravenous pyelogram (IVP). An IVP starts by injecting dye into a vein. Then the kidneys, ureters, bladder, and urethra are observed on an X-ray. Next in the evaluation is a cystoscopy, which required a general anesthetic. This procedure uses a scope to evaluate the inside of the bladder and the urethra. A less-invasive evaluation called a voiding cystogram is used for children twenty-four months and under. A voiding cystogram is a radiological procedure to evaluate the bladder and the urethra. A voiding cystogram is less risky and often does not require sedation.

UTIs are much more common with reflux (urine going back to the kidney from the bladder).

In the past, children with reflux were put on prophylactic antibiotics. This is no longer recommended because giving antibiotics increases the likelihood of developing a drug-resistant infection in the urinary tract. These recommendations are evolving due to complex factors. Some of the factors include age, gender, and whether the UTI was afebrile or febrile (no fever or fever). Today, recommendations include an initial ultrasound of the kidney, ureters, and bladder. In general, prophylactic antibiotics are not used. These guidelines are reviewed and updated.

Fathers in the delivery room

In spite of being a medical student or a physician at the time, I did not see the births of my first five children as it was not the custom at the time. When I first started practicing, only one physician in Denver allowed fathers in the delivery room. This allowance put pressure on the other obstetricians to allow fathers in the delivery room. Gradually, over a number of years, all fathers were allowed in the delivery room if they chose. I was fortunate to see the births of my two youngest children.

Parents watching minor procedures

When I first started practice in 1963, parents were not allowed to watch minor medical procedures such as blood draws, stitches, circumcisions, etc. The rationale for this was based upon concerns including parents fainting, contamination of the surgical field, upsetting the child, making the doctor nervous, etc. This greatly upset some parents because they did not want to be left in the dark and wanted to observe exactly what was being done to their child.

Now parents are given a choice. Allowing parents to be present helps calm the child and the parent. The parent's presence also establishes rapport with the doctor because the parent can see exactly what is being done and the doctor can explain what is happening and why. Many parents express their appreciation for the care provided and realize the skill involved even in executing simple procedures. As my career progressed, I felt more and more comfortable having parents present during these procedures.

Bloxsom Airlock (AL)

A niece of mine was born very prematurely in 1951. She was placed in an AL, which is a sealed chamber with pure oxygen at increased pressure. At that time, it was not known how detrimental oxygen could be to the eyes. Needless to say ALs have not been used for many years. Fortunately, my niece has normal vision.

Syrup of ipecac

Babies put everything into their mouths. At the nine-month checkup, it was common for pediatricians to give parents a small bottle of ipecac. In 1965, the FDA allowed purchase of syrup of ipecac without a prescription. If the baby ingested something toxic, ipecac would induce vomiting. There were a number of problems with this practice. Surprisingly, some toxins are best left in the gastrointestinal tract (GI tract). For example, corrosive substances and hydrocarbons such as petroleum distillates (e.g., gasoline, kerosene, mineral oil, lamp oil, paint thinners) should be left in the intestinal tract. Induced vomiting could also result in aspiration into the lungs (aspiration is when something enters your airway or lungs by accident). Furthermore, studies found ipecac was not very effective in purging the intestinal tract. Finally, giving ipecac at home often delayed the child getting to the emergency room. Today, activated charcoal is given in the emergency room and/or a specific antidote if the ingested toxin has an antidote.

Infant feeding

Ideally, babies should be exclusively breastfed for four to six months, at which time solids are introduced. When I started practice in 1963, babies that were not breastfed were bottle-fed with commercial formulas or evaporated milk formula (evaporated milk, water, and corn syrup). Commercial formulas were introduced in 1867 with the goal of duplicating breast milk. Most of the ingredients of breast milk can be duplicated. However, antibodies and white blood cells found in breast milk cannot be duplicated. Antibodies and white blood cells are important in keeping the baby from getting infections. Breastfeeding has many other advantages—for example, bonding with the mother, statistically less sudden infant death syndrome (SIDS), less infections, etc.

Since 1963, the formula preparation method has greatly changed. Back then, the formula was mixed and put into nursing bottles, and the nipples were loosely applied. The bottles were then placed in a rack, which was submerged in boiling water for twenty-five minutes. Bottles were then stored in the refrigerator and had to be heated before feeding the baby. Today, you take a dishwasher-clean bottle and add several scoops of formula to warm tap water, and the formula is ready to feed to the baby. This process takes only several minutes and is so simple that even fathers are able to make ready a bottle.

Thumb-sucking

Years ago, thumb-sucking was generally discouraged. Some thought it led to dental problems resulting in the need for braces. To prevent thumb-sucking, some dentists put a metal device called a rake behind the upper teeth. An extreme measure was to put the child's arms in casts to prevent the child from putting their thumbs in their mouth. However, it was later determined that many children who never suck their thumbs required braces, and many children who sucked their thumbs did not require braces. Today it is accepted that children just love to suck to calm themselves. I always preferred thumbs over pacifiers. Thumbs are always available. Like pacifiers, they may get dirty, but they don't fall on the floor. Finally, unlike a pacifier, thumbs don't get lost in the middle of the night, requiring parents to wake up and spend time crawling around in the dark trying to find them.

PAUL N. TSCHETTER, MD

Phenobarbital for febrile seizures

In the 1960s, some pediatricians gave parents a prescription for a small bottle of phenobarbital. This was given to patients who had a previous febrile seizure (some children convulse with high fevers). However, in most instances, the child was already convulsing by the time the parents realized the child had a fever. Thus, as a preventive measure, some pediatricians prescribed a daily dose of phenobarbital. Phenobarbital was also prescribed for children who had chronic seizure disorders such as grand mal seizures. Unfortunately, in the 1970s concerns arose about behavioral and cognitive changes in children who were regularly taking phenobarbital for seizure disorders. As a result, phenobarbital is now rarely used to treat seizures.

Concussions

Concussion management in the past was not optimal. Most coaches and athletic trainers thought concussion was not possible unless the child had lost consciousness. However, in many cases, a child can have a concussion without losing consciousness. Due to this misguided belief, many concussed children were never referred to the emergency room or evaluated by a doctor. Even if they were seen, they often got a skull X-ray, which had little value. Fortunately, in recent years great strides have been made in concussion protocol and management. Unfortunately, these strides were made because young athletes died. Now, if an athlete shows the slightest sign of a concussion, either a trainer or physician performs an established sideline concussion evaluation. The athlete must pass each and every step and otherwise demonstrate that he/she is symptom-free before being allowed to continue to participate. In Colorado, a high school athlete may not return to play if the athlete has not passed a concussion protocol evaluation conducted by a physician.

ALMOST FIFTY YEARS' EXPERIENCE AS A PEDIATRICIAN

Screenings

Hearing loss can significantly affect language development and learning. Two to three newborns out of every one thousand have hearing loss. If treatment is started at a very early age, these children have language development comparable to their peers. In the past, many children with hearing loss were not diagnosed until age two or three years when they failed to speak. Unfortunately, by this time, the optimal window for treatment had passed. For quite a while the technology existed for hearing screening. However, it was not until 1992 that a protocol was developed for screening the hearing of newborns. This protocol was the result of a Colorado study using automated auditory brainstem response testing. Around the year 2000, newborn hearing screening became mandatory in Colorado and in many other states. Today all newborns are tested in the newborn nursery, and if they fail that test, follow-ups are scheduled with an audiologist.

Over the years, many additional screening tests have been added. Phenylketonuria (PKU) is a genetic defect. The defect results in decreased metabolism of an amino acid. It may present itself as a musty odor in the breath, skin, and/or urine of the infant. Untreated, PKU can lead to severe intellectual disability, seizures, behavioral problems, and mental disorders. PKU screening was one of the first developed genetic screening tests. Now the list of genetic defect screening has grown to over fifty. Most states now routinely screen for over thirty inherited genetic and metabolic disorders. Many of the conditions screened for can cause intellectual impairment. However, most of them are also treatable if detected shortly after birth. Screening or testing is done by obtaining a very small amount of blood from the newborn using a heel stick. The blood is processed by the state laboratory.

Of all the tests, hypothyroidism is the most commonly positive test. Hypothyroidism, if undetected, can be disastrous. If the baby lacks thyroid hormone, the baby's intelligence will drop significantly to the point of permanent impairment even over the span of just a few months. If detected, treatment starts immediately. The treatment is to provide thyroid hormone for the remainder of the baby's life.

One of the criteria for being tested is that a condition is treatable. At one point, many argued that cystic fibrosis (CF) was not treatable. In the past, a child was not diagnosed for CF until they failed to thrive or had pneumonia. Diagnosing CF at birth allowed for therapies to begin immediately. While these therapies did not cure CF, they greatly increased longevity. Colorado was the first state to test for CF. The advent of drugs to treat CF has significantly prolonged the lifespan and improved the quality of life of CF patients.

Similar to hearing, vision was not tested until about three years of age if at all. Now, most newborns are tested for physical signs of potential vision problems. For example, strabismus (crossed eyes) is a physical sign of vision problems that is treatable.

In addition to hearing and vision testing becoming routine for newborns, our practice added developmental testing starting at birth using the Denver Developmental Screening Test. Our goal was for no child to enter school without normal vision, hearing, and development. Later in years, blood pressure testing was added to the routine. Next was cholesterol. We began checking cholesterol at eleven years and then again at eighteen years of age.

In more recent times, the M-Chat Questionnaire was used to screen for autism between eighteen to twenty-four months. If symptoms of attention deficit hyperactivity disorder (ADHD) are suspected during an annual checkup, the Conners test was used to screen for ADHD. These questionnaires were given to parents and teachers to assess the patient.

Before I left the practice in 2012, we also routinely used questionnaires to screen for anxiety, depression, and suicide (confidential between patient and pediatrician). Around this same time, newborn nurseries started to screen for certain types of congenital heart disease. Over the years, the continued development of screening tests greatly improved care for our patients.

COMMENTS AND OBSERVATIONS BY PATIENTS AND PARENTS

- An eight-year-old young man commented that the waiting room was packed. He then commented, "You must really be raking in the money."
- People often talk louder to people who speak English as their second language. A couple and their infant were obviously from India. I turned to the mother and in a very loud voice asked her where she was from. "Calcutta," she replied. Again, in a really loud voice, I asked the father where he was from. "Connecticut," he replied in perfect English.
- I asked the mother of a five-year-old if her daughter could say all her sounds correctly. The mother replied that the girl had trouble with *S*. She then asked the girl to say the word *exit*.
- The parents of a four-year-old proudly said that she could count to ten. They added that she does not get them in the right order.
- Jennifer took karate so she could protect herself. When I asked how she would use it, she said she would hit the attacker in the stomach. She paused for a moment and then said, "Or a little lower."
- A mother and grandmother were trying to ask intelligent questions during an exam of a newborn. They asked if the newborn boy failed his genetic screen, could he still live in Colorado?

CHAPTER 3

Death

Death is final. Parents are supposed to die before their children. The death of a child is one of the most difficult experiences anyone can face. If a wife dies, the husband is a widower. If a husband dies, the wife is a widow. There is no word to describe the parents who live after a child dies.

Many are surprised that pediatricians deal with death. Unfortunately, pediatricians deal with death too often. Early in my practice, the most common death was that of a premature baby. At that time, if an infant could not breathe on their own, death was inevitable because there were no respirators for premature babies. For many years, I did not keep track of the patients that died. I started to track patient deaths about twenty-five years ago. The following are some of the tragic deaths my patient families experienced.

A father

Think twice! A father went helicopter skiing in Canada and unfortunately was caught in an avalanche. He did not survive and left behind four orphans. Was the risk worth it? Think twice!

ALMOST FIFTY YEARS' EXPERIENCE AS A PEDIATRICIAN

Travis

He was just nine years old and very excited about the load of sand his parents had ordered for his sandbox. The sand was delivered via a dump truck. Travis tragically died when he tunneled into the pile and it collapsed on him. At his service, he was dressed in his baseball uniform holding his glove. Seated in the front row were his baseball buddies. They were all dressed in their uniforms as well.

Bobby

Bobby was a patient for many years. Because he was deaf, he attended a small church school to receive individual help and support from the teachers. He was a good student and a good football player. Like many of his classmates, he went to college. Bobby found the large classes difficult, especially since there was no one to help him. Late one night, when driving down from the west side of the Eisenhower Tunnel, he crashed off the road just before Silverthorne at mile marker 205. His mother said he always wore his seat belt. However, the police said that Bobby was not wearing his seat belt that night.

Three fathers

In a fairly short period of time, three fathers of patients committed suicide. Combined, they left a total of twelve children fatherless. One father hung himself. Another jumped off a four-story parking lot structure. The third drove into the west side divider between the two tunnels just before Idaho Springs. All three had recently been taken off their medications for depression. One was released from the hospital without being prescribed any medication after being admitted for depression. His wife sued the doctor and received a large award to help her four children attend college.

Murder

A week after seeing a female teenage patient, she was murdered at work. A disgruntled teenage male coworker who had been fired returned to the restaurant after hours and killed four employees, including my patient. She had been in two weeks before the shooting and told me that she was earning money to go to college. She was the second oldest of four children. I attended her wake. Her mother pointed out where she had been shot behind her right ear. The perpetrator received the death sentence. Over twenty years later, he was set to be executed. The governor gave him a reprieve and said that the next governor would have to deal with the problem. His sentence was converted to life without parole when Colorado abolished the death penalty.

Leukemia

It was the early 1960s, and children diagnosed with leukemia lived an average of six months. Sidney M. Farber, MD, in Boston was testing drugs that killed cancer cells. The drugs also killed normal cells. Dr. Farber is known as the father of modern chemotherapy.

An eight-year-old patient of mine received several drugs that did not slow the progression of the leukemia. After being admitted to the hospital, he never went home. Every day when I made rounds, I checked on him. He always looked so sad and never spoke a word. It was awful to watch his life slowly fade away.

Dr. Farber continued to try many drugs including combinations of drugs and radiation. Over many years combinations were found that prolonged life. Now 85–90 percent of children diagnosed with leukemia are cured.

Child abuse

It was 6:30 p.m. on a Monday night when the telephone secretary paged me. A family who had just moved from New York had two sick children. Fortunately, an office visit indicated that they just had bad colds.

Several weeks later, a nurse in the office said, "You better take this call." It was a local hospital. The voice on the other end asked if I could sign a death certificate for a child. The death certificate was for one of the children from New York that I had seen on that Monday night. The child arrived at the emergency room severely beaten. Suddenly, I realized that I had read about this in the newspaper.

That evening, I read the story again. The alleged abuser was the mother of another patient of mine. She ran a small daycare in her home and had beaten the child from New York to death with hair clippers. She received a life sentence.

Colon cancer

Several years ago, I learned that a former patient had died of colon cancer at age forty-five. At the time, this seemed very young. After I retired, I was informed that another former patient had died of colon cancer at age nineteen. He had Lynch syndrome, which is hereditary with about one in three hundred people having it. Patients with Lynch syndrome have a much higher risk for colon cancer, anywhere between 20 percent to 80 percent. In comparison, the incidence of colon cancer in the general population is around 4 percent. Individuals with Lynch syndrome should have frequent colonoscopies throughout their life.

Suicides

A former patient in her late twenties bought a shotgun, went to the mountains, and shot herself. Her father, a physician, did not understand why her therapist had no idea of her suicidal mental state or had not prescribed some possible medications. After her death, it was discovered that the therapist was engaged in a romantic relationship with the patient. The therapist didn't refer the young woman to a psychiatrist because she did not want to lose her as a patient.

A nineteen-year-old senior in high school with known depression was on medication and seeing a psychiatrist. One day he did not go to school. When his mother came home from work, she found him dead. I suspected that he had overdosed on his medication. I spoke with his mother several times after his death and gently asked about the autopsy. However, the mother did not want to know the results of the autopsy.

An older former patient had a lot going for himself. After a breakup with his girlfriend, he moved back in with his parents. He started drinking very heavily, and perhaps some street drugs were used. One evening he had a severe argument with his father over his drinking. He finally went to bed, and his father went to wake him up at 5:00 a.m. for his early-morning job. His father found him dead. His father was devastated. The autopsy showed some possible cardiac problems.

A fourteen-year-old boy came home from school and shot himself. He had been under my care since birth, and there were no indications of mental illness. He was an excellent student. I contacted his parents, but they said they had no idea why he shot himself. An aunt was also reluctant to discuss it but did inform me that his most recent grades were not up to his standards.

Auto accident or homicide

Three generations of a family were well-known to me for many years. Growing up, I mowed the grandmother's lawn. After mowing the yard, I would knock on the door, and the grandmother would open the door only enough to stick her hand out with a $1.25. Her daughter later told me that her mother was schizophrenic. The granddaughter was a patient of mine. She was a very happy child with no significant problems. The mother would often write me nice notes thanking me for the care I gave her daughter. Eventually, the granddaughter was married, but it was a bad marriage. One day the mom called, and she told me that her daughter had been killed. Allegedly, she was driving with her husband and somehow fell out of the car. However, this was very suspicious because the husband drove over her twice after she had fallen out of the car. The husband was tried for murder but somehow was acquitted. Fortunately, the mother assumed the care of her daughter's young children.

Electrocution

Years ago a family lost their father when he was working on high-tension electric wires. Their son, a former patient, also became an electrician. Unfortunately, like his father, the son also died when he was electrocuted working on high-tension electric wires.

Cervical cancer

A thirty-three-year-old former patient died of cervical cancer. Her father, a good friend of mine, said it was ironic that she died the very same month that the vaccine to prevent cervical cancer became available. Knowing her lifestyle, it is unlikely that she ever had a Pap smear test.

Auto accidents

Over the years, a number of patients died in auto accidents. Unfortunately, many were caused by drinking. A young college freshman returning from school was intoxicated and drove into a tree. He survived, but his intelligence had been damaged to the extent he could only function at the level of a six-year-old.

A group of young adults, all over age twenty-one, went to a concert. They had rented a hotel room because they would be drinking. The hotel manager asked them to leave because they were noisy. A young lady from the group of five rear-ended another car at ninety miles an hour. The young lady was killed instantly, and a young man in the car, who was a patient of mine, died thirteen days later.

Throughout the almost fifty years of practicing as a pediatrician, I had a number of other patients and parents who died in car accidents. Parents and young drivers alike need to slow down, don't drive under the influence, and always, always, always wear seat belts correctly. I can't emphasize enough that infants, toddlers, and young children need to be securely seated in their car seats or booster seats.

Heartbroken twice

While reading the obituaries one day, a unique name caught my attention. I was certain this person was a former patient of mine. I called the mother, and she shared that her daughter had died of cervical cancer in her early thirties. She also shared that her son had died of leukemia several years earlier.

COMMENTS AND OBSERVATIONS BY PATIENTS AND PARENTS

- Three of my sister's grandchildren came to the office complaining of a rash all over their bodies, but not on their heads. Since my sister has a hot tub, I immediately knew what had caused the rash: a bacterium called Pseudomonas. My sister was horrified to learn that her hot tub was harboring bacteria.
- A few weeks later, another family came in with two children who had the same rash as my sister's grandchildren. They did not have a hot tub, but their neighbor had one, and the children spent a lot of time in this hot tub. After explaining that hot tubs harbor bacteria, the boy said he should have known something was wrong when he noticed the bubbles were brown.
- A little four-year-old girl kept coming in with urinary tract infections (UTIs). After her second or third infection, I ordered an intravenous pyelogram (an X-ray of the urinary tract). The kidneys were normal, but there was a safety pin in her vagina. I explained to the mother that this was the cause of the UTIs. Her comment was that she knew her daughter had not swallowed a safety pin. The knee bone is connected to the thigh bone, the thigh bone is connected to the pelvic bone, but the vagina is not connected to the intestinal tract.

CHAPTER 4

All Doctors Will Become Patients

Over the years, I unfortunately have been diagnosed with several conditions, had several surgeries, and had many other medical procedures. With the exception of one, I didn't consider any of them to be serious. Likewise, with the exception of one doctor, all the physicians involved were great, and this helped a lot. I had five eye surgeries mainly because the doctor botched my cataract surgery and it had to be redone or corrected. I've had fifteen surgeries to remove cancerous skin lesions. In 2000, I had two surgeries: The first was my initial heart surgery (six bypasses). The second was cervical spine surgery. In 2009, I had a hip replacement. About a year later, I had the first of two back surgeries. In 2012, I was diagnosed with Parkinson's disease. Fortunately, it has been well controlled with medication and lots of stretching. I've had a knee surgery and two sinus surgeries. A friend gave me a little book that included a list of twenty things doctors needed to know. I can only remember three of them.

1. All doctors will become patients.
2. Never sleep with someone who does not know CPR.

I will save number 3 for later.

ALMOST FIFTY YEARS' EXPERIENCE AS A PEDIATRICIAN

March 15, 2015, is etched in my memory. This was the day that I admitted to myself that I could no longer read the newspaper. Not even using my special light from the Beyond Vision store. Given current events, I'm probably not missing much.

Three years earlier, my optometrist said he could no longer correct my vision to 20/20. Despite diagnosing me with age-related macular degeneration (AMD) four or five years earlier, he was always able to correct my vision with glasses to 20/20. After receiving this diagnosis, I saw a retinal specialist. He confirmed my AMD diagnosis. AMD is a hereditary disease; my father had AMD, and later my older sister developed AMD.

When I was diagnosed with AMD, my vision was 20/40. After this point, every time my vision was checked, it was worse (20/100, 20/160, 20/200—legally blind). In 2018, I had my semiannual eye exam, and I was unable to read any of the letters on the eye chart. At this time, I could no longer read the TV schedule on our big screen TV. Now when I get an eye examination, the examiner checks my vision by holding up one or two fingers and then asks me how many fingers they are holding up. In September 2020, I was still able to answer correctly. However, at my last examination, I only got one out of four correct, which is worse than if I had just guessed.

When first diagnosed, I could only be corrected to 20/40, I discovered there were some things I could no longer do. I could no longer read the system font on my computer, but I could enlarge document fonts to make them readable. At that time, my best eye was 20/100.

Looking back, after my AMD diagnosis, I had almost a daily decrease in vision. In the summers, my grandchildren compete in swim meets. By 2014, even though I knew which lane they were swimming in, I could barely see them. Faces also became very indistinct, even close up. Mainly just silhouettes. By May 2015, my rapidly declining vision became obvious and concerning to me.

A friend gave me his mother's DaVinci reading machine. You place a document, letter, or book on the machine, then the machine projects the page onto a screen, increasing the font to the point you could read it. For example, I printed emails and could read them by having the machine project them. I appreciated my friend's gesture, but for me, the older machine was user-unfriendly, and I found it difficult to operate. Furthermore, printing the emails was very time-consuming and overall unbeneficial since most emails just need to be deleted.

As my vision deteriorated, driving became more and more difficult. By 2015, I had not driven at night for several years. Near the end, I was limited to driving to church, working out, and having breakfast with a friend. The drive to church and the gym are the same direction and involve only two turns. On August 13, 2015, I drove my last mile. It became obvious by this time that driving was not only a danger to me but more importantly to others and the potential legal liability was huge. I now was totally dependent on others for a ride. My wife became my main source of transportation. While many people do not like driving, I always considered it a special pleasure and miss it greatly.

Since my wife soon grew tired of shuttling me around, I discovered public transportation. In the Denver metro area, public transportation is run by the Regional Transportation District (RTD). RTD has a program called Access-a-Ride. Only qualifying disabled individuals may use this service. RTD tests individuals to determine if they are qualified. A small bus picks you up at your front door and takes you to your destination. When you are finished, a bus comes and takes you home. This is a great service, and the cost could not be beat. With my RTD access pass, I was able to go anywhere RTD goes for $4.50 each way. However, it involves a lot of waiting for the buses. The wait is supposed to be 30 minutes, but I often waited longer. One time after waiting for more than 3 hours, I walked the 2 to 3 miles home. While the service was a definite benefit, it also further drove home the extent of my disability.

In February 2016, it was time to look for a new computer. I could not read my computer even with a magnifying glass. When we were at the Apple Store, I asked if there was a program that could transcribe my dictation. The lady helping us said that a program called Dragon Naturally Speaking did this. However, she said that I didn't need it because the Mac Operating System now was able to transcribe dictation. Oddly, she did not mention that the Mac can also read text (something that I discovered on my own), which I have found invaluable.

A neighbor who also lost his vision turned me on to a store called Beyond Vision. They had a reading machine called DaVinci. Despite my bad experience with the previous reading machine, I gave it a test drive. While it worked like my old machine, it had many additional features and was much more user-friendly. The most important feature is that if you don't feel like reading the enlarged text, you can press a button, and DaVinci reads whatever is on the screen. In addition to the DaVinci, I also purchased a talking scale from Beyond Vision. You simply step onto the scale, and it announces how much you weigh. Unfortunately, Beyond Vision went out of business shortly after I discovered it because the landlord raised their rent too high.

In 2018, a friend told me about a bridge player who wore special glasses that seemed to help her a lot. The name of these glasses is eSight. eSight did not have a Denver office, but I was able to arrange an appointment with a sales representative at a local hotel. The eSight glasses cost $8,500. Fortunately, prior to the appointment, I called the Low Vision Clinic at the ophthalmology department at Anschutz and asked if they had ever heard of these eSight glasses. They had, and in fact they had them in stock. They also had another brand called Iris Vision. After trying on both glasses, there was no comparison; Iris Vision glasses were much better when looking through them. The Iris Vision glasses were also much better in price ($2,500) at less than a third of the eSight glasses.

The Iris Vision glasses are truly amazing. I can now see the faces of my grandchildren, and I can even read with them. The Iris Vision glasses look like I am playing a virtual reality game. The hardware is a Samsung phone programmed by a company in Silicon Valley and came out in 2017. The glasses subsequently released a new application that allows you to take a snapshot of a document and then it will read it out loud. You cannot walk wearing Iris Vision because your balance is thrown off. However, with my new glasses, I can actually see my grandchildren swim if I know in which lane they are swimming.

Overall, while they all take time to operate, the iMac, the DaVinci reading machine, and the Iris Vision glasses have made a dramatic improvement in the quality of my life. I cannot imagine what my life would be like without these wonderful devices. The main downside is that when something goes wrong (and it does), it is very difficult for me to figure out what the problem is without assistance.

Although these devices are extremely helpful, they do not help me accept the difficult reality that my vision will never be better. Nor do they help me with simple, everyday life tasks that most people almost certainly take for granted. Someone with poor vision probably experiences difficulty with some or all the issues that I experience difficulty with or I'm no longer able to perform.

One of the primary impacts of not being able to see is that everything takes so much longer than it used to. Take for example eating. When you can't see the food on your plate well enough to identify it, you eat significantly slower. For most meals, my wife has to identify what is on my plate and cut up my food. If she is not around and all else fails, despite what my mother told me, fingers can be used to eat. At a recent buffet, a friend had to identify what foods were available and helped me fill my plate.

At some point, shopping became impossible. At first, I could not see the prices, and then I was no longer able to identify the items at all. Moving around in the four-level house that I have lived in since 1965 became problematic. The stairs are difficult to see and therefore difficult to use. I have to count all the stairs to make sure that I am on the last step. Because I eventually couldn't see the silverware, unloading the dishwasher became a chore. Getting something out of the refrigerator eventually became difficult because I couldn't see what was in it. While we try to maintain some system, chances are that if I am looking for the ketchup, I won't be able to find it.

You can't or probably shouldn't be mowing your yard when you can't see. As late as 2021, I still mowed the yard using a lawn tractor. It became harder and harder because I became less and less aware of where I had mowed. I last mowed the yard in June of 2021. To this day, I feel that I could still use a chainsaw. My wife, Renee, disagrees and had it shipped off to one of the children's homes after the last time I used it two or three years ago.

Unless carefully tracked, finding simple items is nearly impossible. Keys, glasses, and the TV remote must be placed in the same place or I can't find them without assistance. After the grandchildren have visited, many times it is hard to find the remote. In 2020, it became even more difficult to find things on my desk. As a result, my desk is arranged and maintained a certain way. Performing some routine tasks also proved difficult or at least involved a learning curve. It took me a while to learn how to shave when not being able to use a mirror. Further, even though I know where my pills are, I have difficulty seeing them so my wife has to separate them into specific daily containers.

Maybe some blind individuals, perhaps those that have been blind most of their lives or for a significant portion of their lives, can identify people from their voices. However, for the most part, I cannot. When people come up to me, I don't know who they are for the most part unless they identify themselves. On several occasions I could not even identify my own children. The one advantage is that I never have to be embarrassed because I didn't remember somebody's name because I'm always able to ask, "What is your name?"

For several years, I regularly researched available clinical trials. Coincidentally, my retinal specialist was involved in a large clinical trial. Trial participants had to qualify and sign many consent forms (40–50 pages worth). When I learned that I had qualified, I was ecstatic and thanked God. I began the trial in the summer of 2016. I was optimistic and hopeful that I would receive the clinical drug and not the placebo. The worldwide clinical trial conducted by Roche Pharma cost $3.2 billion. The trial was designed to determine the efficacy of a drug to slow the progression of macular degeneration. Initial results seemed promising.

Once a month, I would go to the Department of Ophthalmology at the CU Medical Center at Anschutz. My vision would be checked, then the doctor would examine my eyes, take photographs of my retinas, and inject the drug into my eye. The injection confirmed to me that I was getting the drug, not the placebo. The eye chart used to check my vision had very large letters (about 15 inches high and 10 inches wide). I still could not read most of the letters even when they brought the eye chart about 3 feet away. My vision was 20/200, or worse, which I later learned that this is the point where you are considered legally blind. Each monthly visit took about two hours.

In November 2018, I was shocked when the clinical trial came to an abrupt halt. At the time, I had completed my 24 months of monthly eye injections and was waiting hopefully for the final results. Because the drug had not had any positive results, the data collected to date was comprehensively analyzed. This analysis concluded that the clinical trial failed to demonstrate that the drug had any value. This was very disappointing, but these types of studies are needed to make progress. Despite the fact that every year plenty of drugs fail at the clinical trial phase, knowing what doesn't work has some value. Another study by the Japanese proved this as well, when a clinical trial based on injecting embryonic stems cells into the eye failed.

In 2017, following a worldwide search, Valeria Canto-Soler, PhD, and all her researchers arrived on the Anschutz Campus. UC Health at University of Colorado used $5 million from the department of ophthalmology and $5 million from the Gates Center to recruit Dr. Canto-Soler. She was joined by her fellow physicians from the Johns Hopkins School of Medicine. Prior to coming to Denver, Dr. Canto-Solar was the director of the Wilmer Eye Institute. The Wilmer Eye Institute focuses on treating blindness in general and AMD specifically because it is the most common cause of blindness in the world.

In 2014, Dr. Canto-Solar and her research group were able to grow a miniature human retina in a petri dish using stem cells. These functioning photoreceptor cells were capable of sensing light. This major breakthrough was three years before Dr. Canto-Soler came to the Anschutz campus. The research group has continued growing retinas since arriving at Anschutz. These small retinas take five to six months to grow. The next phase of the research is to transplant the retinas into little blind pigs. This extremely delicate operation takes a very small piece of the retina and places it in the pig's macula (the macula is where you have your best vision). Since my maculae are totally degenerated (macular degeneration), I have no central vision.

In 2019, my wife, Renee, and I were offered a tour of Dr. Canto-Solar's research lab. Renee saw a small retina when she looked through a microscope. Transplantation into pigs has already started, and hopefully the human transplantation will start in three to five years.

Initially, my vision slowly decreased and then rapidly accelerated until I have almost completely lost my vision. I have suffered from depression nearly my entire life, and the loss of my vision exacerbated my depression. I first noticed my depression when I was in medical school or maybe even before. Unless a person has had depression, it is difficult to describe. My best effort to try would be to put it this way: I would rather have had all the surgeries and procedures described at the start of this chapter than to have suffered from depression for a single day. Medications help but certainly are not a complete solution. Unfortunately, my family has a history of depression. My mother suffered from depression, as well as my two sisters.

I have really come to understand and appreciate the third thing that doctors need to know (from beginning of this chapter). Every day is a blessing!

COMMENTS AND OBSERVATIONS BY PATIENTS AND PARENTS

- "My daughter had a lot of trouble with her asthma last night. I had to give her three breathalyzer treatments" (also known as nebulizer treatments).
- "How old are you?" I asked the patient. "I am four years old," the patient responded. I then asked when they would turn five years old. "On my birthday!"
- Mrs. R said that her son, Jason, had stuck a chocolate mint up his nose. I could not find it and finally concluded that it must have gone down into his stomach. Several weeks later his little sister needed to be seen in the office. While driving to my office, the bright sun made Jason sneeze. Out came the chocolate mint! He promptly picked it up and ate it.

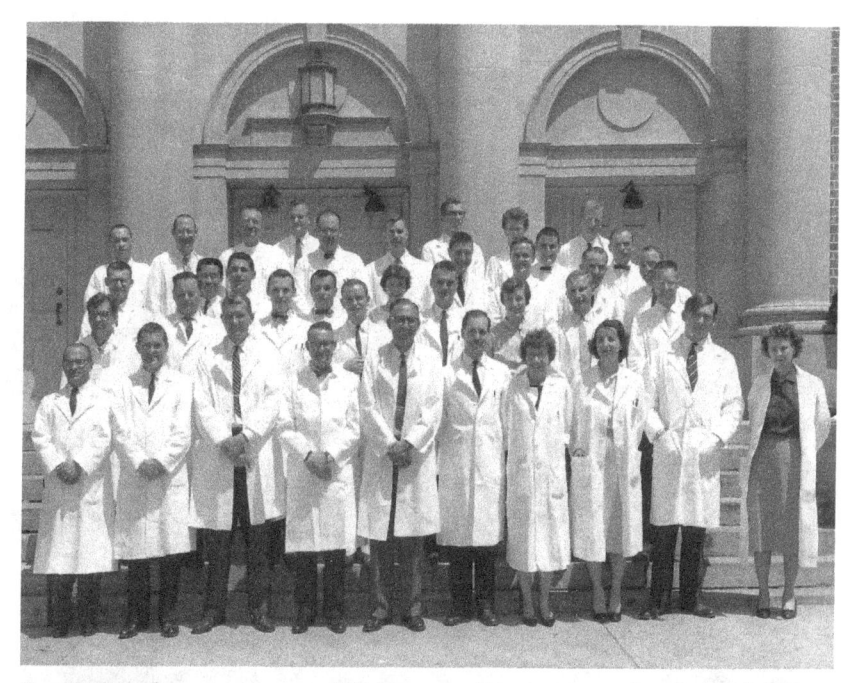

In 1963, there were ten full time pediatric specialists at Children's Hospital (front row). Interns and residents rounded out the staff. Today, the full-time pediatric staff at Children's Hospital Colorado is over 1,000 specialists and researchers.

PAUL N. TSCHETTER, MD

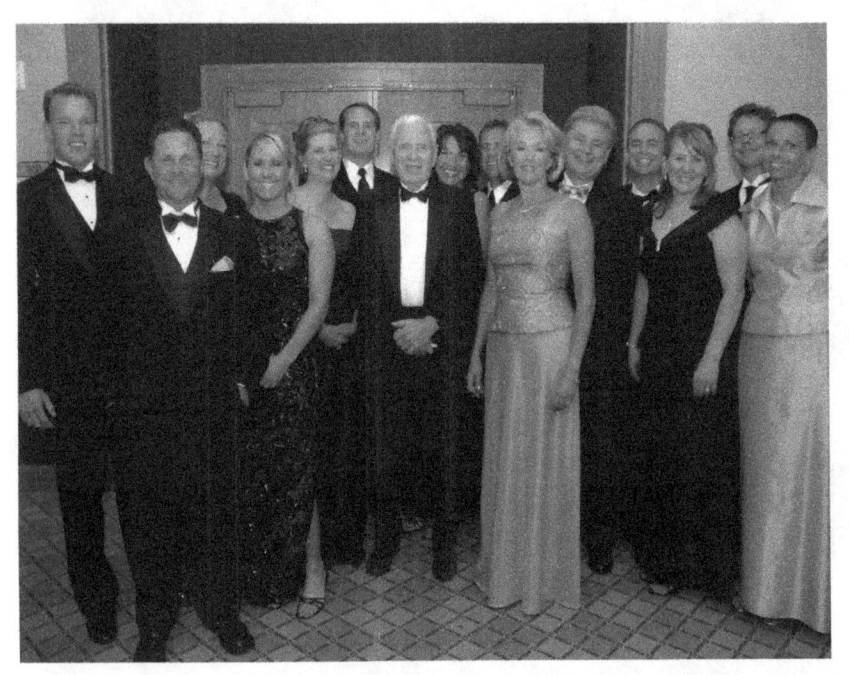

Dr. and Mrs. Tschetter with their children at the Children's Colorado Hospital Gala

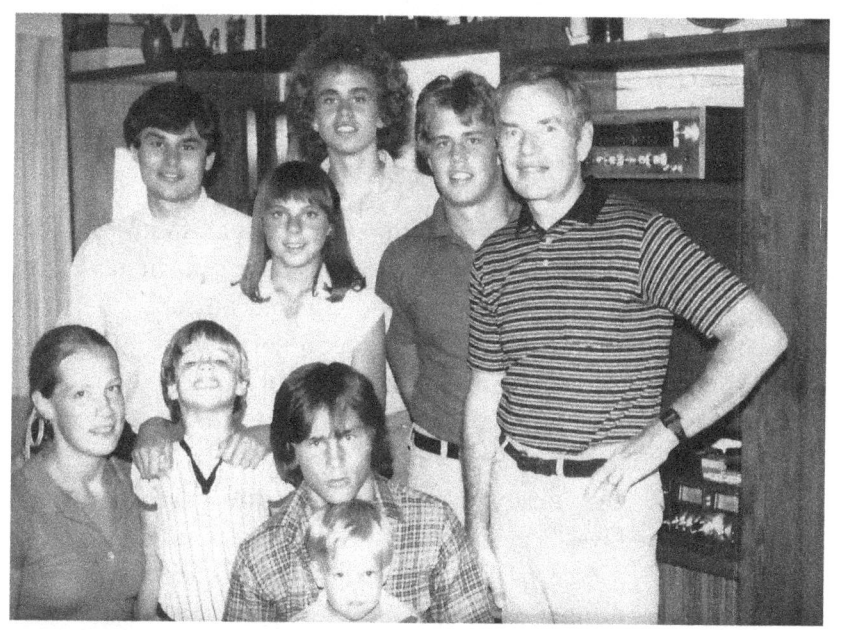

Dr. and Mrs. Tschetter at home with their children. Front row L to R: Renee, Michael, Stephen, Matthew and Dr. Tschetter. Middle row L to R: Nickie and Jon. Back row L to R: David and Mark.

CHAPTER 5

Dignity

"Okay, Paul, scoot your bottom over." With an IV in one arm and wearing a standard hospital gown with one tie at the neck, my back is completely open exposing my wrinkled buttocks. As I try to get over to the catheter table using my one free hand, the gown creeps up to my waist. Luckily the drugs (versed and fentanyl) numb my embarrassment. The two nurses and the male nurse aide make small talk as Paul scoots over.

This is my second angiogram. I don't recall much about my first one because I was heavily sedated. This time I want to watch the monitor as my cardiologist finds my six grafts and checks to be sure they are still open, functional, and not the cause of my chest pain.

My given name is Paul N. Tschetter. However, because my late father's name was also Paul, I have always gone by Nick, which is short for my middle name, Nickolas. The nurses have never met me. They did not introduce themselves, yet they are presumptuous enough to incorrectly address me as Paul. If they came to my office, we would call them Mr. or Mrs. or Ms. If anyone at the office slipped, which occasionally happened, this lack of respect was always discussed at the next staff meeting.

Unfortunately, this situation is not the exception. I had an appointment with my gastroenterologist. While in the waiting room, a nurse aide appeared and said, "Mary, Dr. Lewis is ready to see you." I'm almost surprised that the young nurse aide is wearing jeans (a whole other story). I'm also surprised they don't just say, "Mrs. X, Fred is ready to do your colonoscopy." Anyway, Mary's granddaughter helps her out of the chair, places her hands on her walker, and helps her through the door. The next steps will be disrobing, putting on the gown with one tie, and having someone stick a scope up her colon. Not the most dignified procedure. Given this, you would think that the doctor's office could at least address her respectfully as Mrs. X.

Contrast my experience with my hip surgery anesthesiologist. "Dr. Tschetter, you have several options for anesthesia. You could have a general like you had for your right hip or a local." The young anesthetist speaking was a former patient of mine. He along with his twin brother wrestled in high school. I met him because I was the team physician for thirty-two years. I always appreciated Dr. David Nowick. He is extremely professional and his care is outstanding. Unfortunately, some of the hospital nurses and aides still called me hon, sweetheart, and Paul.

Even after decades in practice, I still refer to the doctors that I trained under as doctor followed by their last name, as in Dr. Smith. I feel strongly that the older doctors in the community deserve my respect. Our staff always called me Dr. Tschetter. I always wanted the staff to have this same level of respect for my younger associates. They were to be addressed by their title and surname, especially in front of patients. I felt that patients didn't want their crying 18-month-old with a 104-degree fever to be evaluated by Hoke or Julie, but rather by Dr. Stapp or Dr. Deckerman. I believe projecting a professional atmosphere is important.

UC Health at University of Colorado asks patients how they would like to be addressed. This information is put on their medical chart, and that is how doctors, nurses and other personnel address them. Some people argue that this violates HIPAA (Health Insurance Portability and Accountability Act) because it discloses "personally identifiable information" about a patient. In my experience, this is absurd because all the medical personnel involved are treating the patient. Further, HIPAA is loosely enforced and in some instances even farcical. For example, when I was practicing, if I wanted to see the results of a patient's X-ray, I would log into Children's Hospital's radiology department. Once logged in, I would see the names of all persons who had imaging that day, even though these were not my patients. Another example, over 212 people accessed a teenager's medical records within 24 hours of her committing suicide at Children's Hospital. The unauthorized access included 12 doctors. While everyone was disciplined, the damage was done.

Being ill is difficult and frightening both for those of us with medical sophistication and those without. Patients have no choice other than to put their trust into the hands of their doctors and those who assist them. Treating persons with dignity when they are sick goes a long way. The medical community needs to set the standard by treating every patient with dignity. When medical professionals call people they don't know by their first name, they are treating them like a child, dehumanizing them, and patronizing them.

Likewise, in some pediatric practices, you hear the doctors and staff calling mothers *mom*. In my opinion, this is most disrespectful. Mothers should be addressed by their surname. After all, the mothers don't call the physician *doc*.

I don't think I am old-fashioned or a fuddy-duddy. Studies have shown that people still prefer to be called by their surname. People also strongly prefer appropriate dress by medical personnel. Overall in my experience, a patient's confidence is increased when healthcare providers treat them with dignity and respect.

COMMENTS AND OBSERVATIONS BY PATIENTS AND PARENTS

- I asked the mother of a two-year-old if he could scribble. "Yes, but not very well," she replied.
- The little eighteen-month-old would not hold still as I was trying to check his abdomen. The mother asked if she could help, and I said "Yes, hold his legs." She replied, "His hind legs?"

CHAPTER 6

Short Stories

Elizabeth and James Christopher

A grandfather who is a pediatrician encounters cases that are close to home. Elizabeth was born to my son and daughter-in-law in 2010. Almost immediately she was having difficulty breathing. Swedish Hospital immediately transferred her to the Neonatal Intensive Care Unit (NICU). Based on Elizabeth's condition, she was placed on a ventilator and intravenous fluids were given along with surfactant to mature her lungs. This was very frightening. Within twenty-four hours, her breathing was normal. It was a miracle and a real blessing!

James Christopher is the sixth child of my son and daughter-in-law. When my daughter-in-law had her twenty-three-week checkup, her blood pressure was found to be very high. She was airlifted to University Hospital Colorado, where she was confined to bed rest.

At twenty-seven weeks gestation, my daughter-in-law went into labor, and James was delivered weighing 845 grams (one pound, fourteen ounces). He too received surfactant to mature his lungs. He remained in the hospital for three months.

When James Christopher was two and a half years old, we started to believe his development might be okay. At his four-year checkup, his development was felt to be pretty much on target. Then the five-year checkup came about, and James had an excellent vocabulary. He was still very small but continued to grow. What a blessing!

Stomachache detective

At nine o'clock in the morning, a nurse asked me if I could see a child with a bad stomachache before my first checkup. A twelve-year-old boy had woken at four in the morning complaining of stomach pain around his belly button. Other questions were negative. He had no diarrhea, vomiting, fever, back pain, pain with urination, sore throat, etc. No one else in the family was sick. He had eaten a good breakfast, and on examination his abdomen was completely soft. His blood count and urinalysis were normal. Generally, the closer the pain is to the belly button, the less likely it is to be serious. It was reasonable to observe him at home.

As his mother was leaving, she said, "Can you note in all the children's records that my husband got shot in the abdomen yesterday?" The father, who was a police detective, responded to a robbery. The robber was pointing a shotgun at the detective when the detective's gun jammed. The father's partner shot the robber. When the robber was falling forward, his gun went off. The buckshot from the robber's shotgun ricocheted off the ground and hit the father in the abdomen. Based on this, I concluded that there was a direct connection between the boy's abdominal pain and his father being shot in the stomach. When I told the mother, she only shrugged. I sent the boy home feeling quite confident that he was just fine.

Croup

When I first started practicing medicine in the early 1960s, hospitals did not staff emergency rooms with physicians. Night or day, if a patient went to an emergency room, you had to go see the patient. One time a nurse called from Porter Hospital in Denver at about 3:30 a.m. She said a patient of mine was having trouble breathing and seemed in distress. I got into my Volkswagen Bug and made the ten-minute trip to Porter Hospital's emergency room.

Tyler's fever was 104 degrees, and he seemed very uncomfortable. I carefully examined his throat first. There was a very *red cherry* on his epiglottis. I had never seen this before, but I immediately knew he had acute epiglottitis. This could advance rapidly to total breathing obstruction. Given there weren't any physicians at Porter Hospital who could perform a tracheotomy, I knew I needed to get Tyler to Children's Hospital, where he could have a tracheotomy or be intubated. Children's Hospital was fifteen minutes away. Tyler, his mother, and I got into my Volkswagen and headed north to Children's Hospital Denver. We had called ahead to the emergency room, and an anesthesiologist was waiting for us. Tyler was quickly intubated. He could breathe again thanks to being intubated. This was the only case of acute epiglottitis I saw in my forty-nine years of practice. Several years later, the *Haemophilus influenzae* type b (Hib) vaccine came out for the bacteria that causes acute epiglottitis.

Joey

Similar to the lack of ER doctors, there were also no nurse practitioners to attend high-risk deliveries. Pediatricians had to attend all high-risk deliveries. During one said delivery, an obstetrician called me and asked me to attend a delivery because the baby was premature. When the baby was born, he was blue and had a weak pulse. One minute after birth, his APGAR* score was 1. Healthy newborns usually have an APGAR score of 7 to 10. Infants with a score of 0 to 3 have severely depressed vital signs and are at great risk of dying unless actively resuscitated. We started resuscitation, and I intubated him. At five minutes, his APGAR score was still 1. Desperately, I gave him a caffeine injection, and he started to breathe, his pulse increased, his color improved, and he started to move his arms and legs. He was transferred to The Children's Hospital's Neonatal Intensive Care Unit (NICU).

The next morning on rounds, the chief neonatologist told me that he would not have resuscitated a child with an APGAR score of 1 at 5 minutes because the child probably would have suffered brain damage. I cared for Joey all the way through high school. He was a solid B student and a great baseball player. After he completed college, I unfortunately lost track of him.

*Developed in 1952 by Virginia Apgar, MD, an anesthesiologist at Columbia University. The test measures a baby's color, reflexes, heart rate, muscle tone, and respiratory ability after birth. This test allows physicians to better treat newborns who may need additional medical attention.

Illegal drugs don't always kill you, but they can

One Tuesday morning at 10:00 a.m., the Swedish Hospital Intensive Care Unit (ICU) called me. A patient of mine had been airlifted from Steamboat Springs to Denver. He was on life support. He had consumed an unknown amount of alcohol combined with marijuana and crack cocaine. His roommate found him in a coma, and he never regained consciousness. After three days, he was declared brain dead and removed from life support. I attended his memorial. This service was very emotional for me as he was the same age and had the same name as our youngest son, Matthew.

The following fall I was doing a checkup on his younger brother. "Do you still attend Highlands Ranch High School?" I asked. He said he was attending a special high school in the mountains. This high school is for adolescents who use drugs. I could not fathom that he was also an addict after his brother died from a drug overdose. Months later, a nurse from Health One Hospital ICU in Aurora called. Tragically and heartbreakingly, the story repeated. After graduating from high school the previous spring, Richard came home for Christmas break. He and his friends were doing drugs, and he took three different illicit drugs. After he lapsed into a coma, his friends thought the cold night air might help him. Because his friends thought they would get into trouble for also using illegal drugs, his friends were hesitant and reluctant to take him to the emergency room. After realizing the cold air would not revive him, they finally called 911. When I arrived at the hospital, Richard was in the ICU on life support. After a week passed, his ICU physician called a meeting of all his doctors. We decided to give him another three weeks because all his organs were functioning well. At thirty days, Richard's life support was removed. His pulse remained strong, but he could not maintain his breathing. Sadly, six hours later he died.

I am certain that neither of these young men wanted to die. However, when experimenting with drugs, most users never think about the unnecessary chance they take because any dose could be lethal. So tragic and so sad, the loss of life too soon, I know how this loss impacted me, but I can't begin to imagine how unbearably sad the loss was for the family.

Broken bones

Five weeks after beginning practice, the phone rang on a Saturday afternoon. A mother said she was having a hard time keeping her eighteen-month-old awake and that the toddler had fallen from her highchair that morning and bumped her head. Upon examination, I could not arouse the toddler and noted a very slow pulse and an elevated blood pressure. These signs indicated an increase in intracranial pressure. In 1963, CT scans and MRIs did not exist to assist in defining the problem. The neurosurgical consultant suggested a skull X-ray, which showed a skull fracture. The little girl was taken to the operating room. I gave her oxygen as she needed no anesthesia since she was in a coma. The neurosurgeon opened her skull and found an acute epidural bleed. He stopped the bleeding, the blood clot was removed, and the little girl regained consciousness. The neurosurgeon assured the mother that she would be fine. Tragically, a few hours later, she bled out and died. The autopsy revealed that she had blue sclera, which is a diagnostic indicator for osteogenesis imperfecta. Additionally, X-rays also revealed several old fractures in various stages of healing, which confirmed the final diagnosis of osteogenesis imperfecta (brittle bone disease). With this condition, a child's bones break extremely easily. The term literally means "bone that is imperfectly made from the beginning of life."

ALMOST FIFTY YEARS' EXPERIENCE AS A PEDIATRICIAN

Theresa

An eleven-month-old female was brought in because she wasn't moving her limbs. She had well over twenty fractures. The child abuse team was called to evaluate her case. Because she was not in daycare, her parents were the only suspects. The emergency room attending physician was consulted and noted that she had blue sclera. The diagnosis was not child abuse, but osteogenesis imperfecta (brittle bone disease). Her bones were so brittle that the parents could cause a fracture with the simple act of changing her diaper. By the age of one year, my records indicated she probably had over one hundred fractures. As time went on, metal rods were placed in all her long bones—all the bones of the arms and legs. Theresa never walked and was confined to a wheelchair. She also had severe scoliosis. I never saw Theresa when she wasn't smiling.

Theresa graduated from high school with high honors. The last time I heard from her mother, she was a student at Colorado State University studying to earn a biomedical science degree.

Battered child

It was 1963, my intern and I had a new admission. She was referred to Colorado General Hospital Department of Pediatrics by a southeast Denver pediatrician. The chief concern for the patient was an enlarged head on the growth chart. Her medical history noted that the fifteen-month-old had been hospitalized at twelve months of age with a broken femur. The mother explained that she had caught her leg in the slats of her crib. Examination showed the child had a large head. The circumference was well over the ninetieth percentile. Retinal hemorrhages were also found. Skull X-rays showed she had a skull fracture. The neurosurgical consultant diagnosed a subdural hematoma (blood clot on the brain). This accounted for her growing head size. The hematoma was drained.

Child abuse was suspected. The pregnancy was unplanned, and the father was suspected to be the abuser. He seemed unstable and reportedly had recently shot a dog that was running across his newly seeded lawn. The attending physician decided that my intern and I should meet with the father and confront him with what we suspected. We were certain that he would pull out a gun and shoot us. However, in short order, we realized he was a very caring father.

Further discussion with the mother revealed that she had not wanted this child. She had broken the little girl's leg and had hit her head with a blunt object. The mother was the daughter of a local chief of police who had abused his daughter (the mother). This case was written up by Dr. C. Henry Kempe, MD, and published in the Journal of the American Medical Association (JAMA). Dr. Kemp had surveyed a number of law enforcement agencies and found there were many cases of children dying under unexplained or suspicious circumstances in the population at large. The title of the article is "The Battered Child Syndrome." This is where the term *battered child* came from.

RJ, kidney failure

The year I was chief resident at Colorado General Hospital, the head of the Department of Pediatrics, C. Henry Kempe, MD, went on sabbatical for one year. While small in physical stature, Dr. Kempe's brilliance loomed large in the Denver medical family. Dr. Kempe was a full professor at age thirty-three. Even though he ruled with an iron hand, he was loved by the community of pediatricians.

Dr. Kempe had a large impact on pediatric patient RJ's life. RJ had end-stage renal failure. He would come to the emergency room in renal failure and was resuscitated many times. Just before Dr. Kempe left on his sabbatical, he called me to his office and said, "I expect RJ to be here when I return." During Dr. Kempe's absence, RJ was the first child in Denver to receive a kidney transplant. RJ was successfully given a kidney from his mother.

About ten years later, I ran into RJ as I came out of Porter Hospital. He was doing well, and he had a successful second transplant.

ALMOST FIFTY YEARS' EXPERIENCE AS A PEDIATRICIAN

Nate

One Sunday afternoon, I received a long-distance call from Nebraska from a couple whose two-year-old I had cared for before they moved. They now also had a nine-month-old baby, Nate, and asked if I could see him as they were going to be visiting family in Denver. They were concerned about the baby's vision.

At my office, I could not get the baby to track objects or follow a light. Children nine months of age should be able to do both. Nate also failed his motor development milestones. He could barely support his head, and he could not sit. I referred him to The Children's Hospital in Denver. An excellent pediatric ophthalmologist also could not determine if Nate could see. This was 1965, and sophisticated tests to check vision were not available. We assumed he was blind.

Nate's motor development was slow, and he had no language before three years of age. As his language development progressed, much of it was echolalia (unsolicited repetition of vocalizations made by another person). His father was a sports announcer, and much of what Nate said were things he heard his father say on the radio:

> He is going to score!
> The fans are screaming!
> It is fourth down.
> The bases are loaded.

Everyone involved with Nate's care met in Arapahoe County at Developmental Pathways to discuss Nate's treatment plan. During the meeting, one of Nate's developmental therapists gave him a block and asked him if it was red. Because Nate only answered yes or no correctly 50 percent of the time, we were completely taken back when the therapist asserted that he could tell his colors based on this test.

Nate loved to play putt-putt golf. He would always make a hole in one. He would hit the ball, and a family member would drop another ball in the cup. Nathan was very happy when he heard the ball falling into the cup. Nate was about thirty years old when I learned that he had died of cancer. After the service, I spoke with his parents. Nate had surgery and was put on chemotherapy. He did not understand what the medicine was for, but he knew it made him very sick. For this reason, the chemotherapy was discontinued. Nate loved Glenn Miller, and at the conclusion of his service the strains of "In the Mood" could be heard filling the chapel.

Developmental delays (mental retardation)

In recent years, the preferred term for *mental retardation* was changed to *developmental delays*. A consensus emerged that mental retardation has a negative connotation. While not advocating for the retention of mental retardation, we can and should do better than developmental delays. Developmental delay means the child can develop life's necessary abilities over time. In other words, the child will develop as expected and similar to children without developmental delays, simply because the child has only been delayed.

My experience conclusively showed this not to be the case. I never saw a developmentally delayed child catch up to normal children. Based on this, the term *developmentally challenged* would be better than developmentally delayed. Regardless of the terminology, the reality of dealing with this condition is extremely difficult and challenging for all involved.

While terminology needs to be improved, the diagnosis of developmental related issues has greatly improved from when I started practicing medicine. During my training, a neurologist that I trained with would wait until a child was nine to twelve months old before determining with certainty that the child was delayed. Today, pediatricians attempt to pursue diagnosis at the first sign of any delayed development. For example, an infant should be able to raise her head off a mat by three months. If she can't do this, physical therapy is started immediately. Similarly, because a Down syndrome baby is known to be delayed at birth, therapy is also started immediately.

ALMOST FIFTY YEARS' EXPERIENCE AS A PEDIATRICIAN

A very sad experience

Very early in my career, one appointment with a family involved a delayed child. At nine months of age, the child did not have a social smile. He could not roll over. Both of these milestones indicate developmental abnormalities. He also had head lag. Head lag during a standard neurological exam indicates developmental issues as well. (A child's head lags if the neck doesn't flex to keep the head upright when the child is pulled up by their arms.) I told the family as gently as I could that their little boy was mentally retarded. They had a number of questions. I answered them honestly and as compassionately as I could. Regardless, I was the messenger with bad news.

Because they did not like this news, they transferred to a different pediatrician shortly after the appointment. Even though I was no longer the boy's doctor, I continued to hear about the child through mutual friends. The first news was that the family had enrolled the child in a Doman-Delacato program in Philadelphia.

The father was a teacher and coach at a local high school. He enlisted several high school clubs to raise money for travel and treatment. Despite any demonstrable progress according to the reports I received, the mother reported unbelievable success with the patterning. She reported that her son won an award for crawling the furthest and that he completed algebra and was ready for geometry. I was terribly saddened at the time to hear this because it was not possible to be true.

A few years later I saw him at a high school football event in Cherry Hills. His body was very rigid as the father held him. He was totally unresponsive to the environment and the people at the event. Several years later I learned that the father had died of a sudden heart attack in his backyard after a run. I was also told that social services investigated the home and the mother was accused of child abuse and drug use. Based on this, social services removed him and all the other children from the home.

Wikipedia describes Doman-Delacato as a treatment modality of patterning and was developed in the 1960s by Glenn Doman and Carl Delacato.

Psychomotor patterning, rarely referred to as the Doman-Delacato technique, is a pseudoscientific approach to the treatment of intellectual disabilities, brain injury, learning disabilities, and other cognitive diseases. The treatment is based on the largely discredited hypothesis that ontogeny recapitulates phylogeny. The method assumes that intellectual disabilities results from the failure of an individual to develop properly through the phylogenetic stages, and treatment primarily focuses on non-invasive physical therapy in each of these stages. In one such stage, the homolateral stage, a healthy child typically crawls by turning the head to one side while extending the arm and leg of the opposite side. The patterning treatment is applied to those unable to perform this motion, and involves passive intervention by 4–5 adults who assists the child in an effort to impose or induce the proper pattern onto the central nervous system. The therapy normally lasts for 5 minutes and is repeated at least 4 times a day. Full treatment programs typically contain a range of exercises combined with sensory stimulation, breathing exercises designed to increase oxygen flow to the brain, and systematic restriction and facilitation designed to promote hemispheric dominance.

Richard

I was seeing Richard (age four years) as a new patient. As I entered the room, the mother said, "Never say that Richard should be placed in an institution or group home." I agreed. A developmental exam placed him at about four *months*. The parents moved into a school district that had a good reputation for handicap programs. Richard received physical therapy, occupational therapy, and speech therapy. (Colorado has passed legislation that states a child with the worst handicaps receive the most services from school districts. Because of Richard's condition, his mom lobbied the Colorado General Assembly to fund service programs for handicapped children.)

As the years went by, I continued to see Richard for his checkups and illnesses. Developmentally he had made no progress. Richard was about ten years old when his father and brother moved out of the home and the parents got a divorce. Unfortunately, this is all too common with families who have a handicapped child. When Richard was about fourteen years old, his mother told me she had placed him in a residential home for the handicapped.

Bobby

Bobby was an active toddler. When he was six years old, his parents were concerned about his vision. An ophthalmologist saw him but could not test him because Bobby was uncooperative. Bobby's teacher was concerned that he was hyperactive and would not pay attention. The Conners scale indicated that he had Attention Deficit Hyperactivity Disorder (ADHD). After being placed on medication, there was some improvement. He saw the ophthalmologist again, and it was determined that he was blind. He was doing very poorly in school and seemed to sleep a lot. A neurologist was consulted, and he was diagnosed with a very rare genetic disorder called Batten Disease. This disease is a progressive rare central nervous system disease. It can cause seizures, vision loss, and cognitive and neurological issues. It is fatal.

Eventually Bobby became incontinent and spent most of his time in bed. The parents chose to keep him at home and did not want any heroics if he was dying. A do-not-resuscitate (DNR) form was completed. A copy was sent to the local fire department. Bobby died peacefully at home at age seventeen. His loving family was with him to the end. His mother did not call 911 until he had been dead for some time. She did not want to take a chance that some well-meaning emergency medical technician would try to resuscitate him.

Cody F.

I first met Cody when he was about eight years old. He had the worst case of Attention Deficit Hyperactivity Disorder (ADHD) I had seen. The first time I saw him, he was climbing the wall in between the waiting room seating area and the play area. His mother said he had recently set fire to his mattress.

In the classroom, his teacher reported he required 50 percent of her classroom/teaching time. After each appointment, before he left the office, I always had him empty his pockets of syringes and other medical implements.

His father was an alcoholic who refused to medicate his son. Eventually the father relented. Still, Cody had his tendencies. One day he was chasing a ball that went into the street. He stopped, started at the curb, and ran into the street to get the ball. He was hit by a car and fractured his femur.

Later in life, he was put into a residential treatment facility. To get a mattress, a patient had to earn points. Cody almost always slept on the floor. A number of years later, I read a newspaper article, "Washing Machine Bandit." Cody would go into apartment complex laundry facilities and take apart the machines to get the money. However, he always neatly lay the parts out for the repair man.

Darlene and James

A young girl and her little brother came in for checkups. She was six years old, and he was four years old. It was obvious something was wrong. The mother explained that they were both mentally retarded. The boy was worse than his sister. Their previous pediatrician had made this diagnosis without any tests or evaluations being completed. This was in the mid-1960s, and the main question was should they stay at home or be placed at Ridge Home (a facility for the mentally retarded). The mother, a nurse, said they were very easy to care for and planned for them to continue to live at home. As teenagers, they worked at a pet store. James swept the floors and occasionally did some stocking. Darlene worked at the cash register, but each time she checked someone out she had to be told how to do it again.

Several years after they left my care, the mother called and told me that they had been diagnosed with Fragile X syndrome. According to the US National Library of Medicine, Fragile X syndrome is a genetic condition that causes a range of developmental problems including learning disabilities and cognitive impairment. Their diagnosis did not exist when I was seeing them in the 1960s. The gene for Fragile X was found in 1991. As of a few years ago, the mother informed me that they were still living at home.

Henry and Angela

As a physician, it is always a compliment when a friend or colleague brings their children to you. The father of these children was a classmate of mine from high school.

Henry was about eighteen months old, and Angela about six months old when I first saw them. Henry could speak some words and was learning to walk. I thought he had mild spastic diplegia cerebral palsy. I sent him to a pediatric neurologist who concurred with my diagnosis and sent him to physical therapy. The physical therapist thought he might be able to walk with crutches. Over the next few months, it became obvious that his speech was regressing. Every time he came to the office, I would ask him to show me how he used his crutches. It seemed there was always some reason that he was not willing to try. A few months later his parents and I agreed that his language and motor development were regressing. The neurologist saw him again and a urine test showed that he had a rare recessive disease called metachromatic leukodystrophy (MLD). His sister, Angela, who appeared totally normal up to that point in time, was tested and diagnosed with the same condition. The mother-in-law was convinced that the condition was caused because the mother of Angela and Henry did not keep a clean house. Several years later both children died quietly at home. Angela passed before Henry. May they rest in peace.

Caring for a handicapped child

Families with a handicapped child have a very difficult task. Seeing these families has often made me wonder if I would be able to care for a handicapped child. Many require care twenty-four hours a day. This care includes charting and monitoring medications and oxygen levels. Positioning and changing the child to avoid bedsores. Dealing with feeding issues including using feeding tubes. Scheduling and attending doctor appointments, physical therapy, occupational therapy, and speech therapy. Because many of these children cannot use a traditional car seat, transportation can be difficult. Finding someone to care for a handicapped child is difficult because that person requires the same skills the parents have learned. Often times parents take turns caring for the child, but this prevents them from spending time together. Frequently, as a child becomes older, the parents must have ramps built to get the child in and out of the house. Many routine child care activities such as bathing can be very difficult. Given these enormous challenges, I was always very impressed to see how well these handicapped children were cared for when they came to the office. They were clean and did not have diaper rashes or bed sores. The parents and siblings often told me all the lessons that they had learned from the child. These families had compassion and empathy for the handicapped child. They also had great understanding and appreciation for other handicapped individuals and their families. Sometimes a handicapped child died, and when they did, they were sorely missed by their family. Ironically, there is no word or label to describe those left behind when a child dies, like a widow or widower.

Leonard

It was Sunday morning rounds and urgent office visits were over. Porter Hospital emergency room called. A teenage patient was there with multiple facial lacerations. In those days, there were no emergency room physicians so I drove in to care for him. Reportedly, he had fallen into a pile of bricks and cut up his face. It took over two hours to repair all the lacerations. Halfway through the procedure, some police officers arrived. He had not fallen into a pile of bricks. He and several friends had stolen a car and were joyriding. He crashed the car and went through the windshield—seat belts were not used at that time. After I finished sewing the lacerations, the police put a pair of handcuffs on him and then walked him to their squad car. Many years later, I saw Leonard on TV speaking for his family. I recognized him by the scar on his right cheek. Leonard's father had been stabbed and robbed while walking from his office to his car. He had been taken to the emergency room but later died from severe blood loss. I called the family and spoke with Leonard's sister. I was glad to hear that all four of the children were doing well and had not gotten into any further trouble. She also shared that her mother was not doing well as she had Alzheimer's disease.

Cystic fibrosis

In the 1960s, if you were born with cystic fibrosis (CF), it was a death sentence. Cystic fibrosis was eventually diagnosed when children failed to thrive and developed pneumonia. A medical school classmate had a cousin with CF. She lived to age seventeen and was one of the oldest surviving people with CF. Colorado was one of the first states to screen newborns for CF. Knowing the diagnosis, treatment could be started immediately and severe malnutrition could be minimized.

Decades later, a patient of mine was diagnosed with CF at birth. As a teenager, he played sports and was a weightlifter. He even obtained a hockey scholarship to play for the University of Denver. Years earlier, it would have been unheard of for somebody diagnosed with CF to function in society at such a high level.

My niece moved to Denver with her three sons. She was pregnant at the time. The oldest boy developed nasal polyps, so I referred him to an ears, nose and throat specialist (ENT). The ENT called me and said that even though the boy seemed very healthy, we should screen him for CF. The test came back positive. He was born in Pennsylvania, and they did not screen for CF at birth. My niece delivered her fourth son, and he tested positive for CF. After these positive tests, it took her a long time to have the other two boys tested, but fortunately they both tested negative.

Teenagers have a hard time doing their complex CF treatments consistently as they have more important things to do. Her oldest son questioned whether he should even go to college as he said the average person with CF lives to age thirty-seven. I pointed out to him that every day that goes by the treatments will improve. Her oldest boy completed college as an aeronautical engineer. He is married and has an engineering job with an aerospace company. The youngest boy received a full scholarship to college, and he also became an engineer.

Now there is a drug that treats certain genetic types of CF. It costs about three hundred thousand dollars per year.

A lot of the treatment burden is placed upon the patient as they get older.

Ricky

It was 1963, and it was my second weekend to cover the practice. A newborn patient of ours needed an exchange transfusion (to have his blood exchanged) because he had a high bilirubin count. The patient's Rh incompatibility with his mother's blood was causing the high bilirubin (mom was Rh negative and the infant was Rh positive). Bilirubin is the product of red blood cells being broken down. Our liver removes bilirubin as it is produced. Because infants have immature livers, they cannot remove bilirubin as fast as it is produced. The goal of an exchange transfusion is to first lower the bilirubin level. The second goal is to remove the antibodies the mother has produced against the baby's red blood cells. Hopefully, this will keep the bilirubin count under twenty.

High bilirubin counts can create a condition called kernicterus. Kernicterus is caused when the bilirubin gets into the brain and can cause permanent damage. The most common effects are mental retardation and cerebral palsy (CP). The exchange transfusion can be done by removing small amounts of the baby's blood and infusing an equal amount of donor blood. This process is done many times, and it reduces the bilirubin count and antibodies.

While I was doing the exchange transfusion, a doctor from a small town in southern Colorado called me about an infant named Ricky. Because Ricky had a very high bilirubin level, the doctor was sending Ricky to Children's Hospital in Denver for an exchange transfusion. Meanwhile, my patient with the Rh incompatibility was successfully treated. Ricky was not so fortunate. The small-town physician who had referred Ricky was not familiar with ABO incompatibility. When Ricky arrived at Children's Hospital in Denver, his bilirubin count was fifty-six. This was unprecedented. After three exchange transfusions, his bilirubin level was still thirty-two. I continued to see Ricky for many years for an annual evaluation. He was deaf and mentally retarded.

When a mother and an infant are blood-type incompatible, red blood cells may get into the mother's blood from the baby. The mother's body then makes antibodies against these red blood cells from the baby. In turn, this breaks down the baby's red blood cells, and the product is called bilirubin. (In the past, incompatibility between the mother's Rh factor and the baby's Rh factor was the most common cause of elevated bilirubin in the infant.) The antibodies then return to the baby and break the baby's red blood cells down at a faster rate.

At some point, it was discovered that an ABO blood type incompatibility could also elevate bilirubin levels. An ABO incompatibility results when the mother has O blood type and the baby has type A, B, or AB blood type. In the past, when Rh incompatibility was the most common cause of elevated bilirubin, known as hyperbilirubinemia, an exchange transfusion was performed if the bilirubin was over twenty. Now if the mother is Rh negative, she can receive a shot of RhoGAM that prevents her from making antibodies against her baby's Rh positive red blood cells. For this reason, Rh incompatibility has become almost nonexistent. Now, ABO incompatibility is more common, but usually not as severe as Rh incompatibility.

The ABO incompatibility factor was not as serious as the Rh factor. However, it could result in jaundice. If the jaundice became severe enough, ABO babies had exchange transfusions.

In the 1960s, a pediatrician discovered that natural lighting significantly reduced jaundice in babies. In 1968, Jerold F. Lucey, MD, published a controlled study documenting that babies hospitalized in nurseries with windows (exposed to natural sunlight) had lower levels of bilirubin compared to babies hospitalized in nurseries without windows. Because phototherapy is now widely used to treat jaundice, exchange transfusions are rarely needed.

Bush adoption

Four years after adopting a little girl, a family adopted a boy infant. Randy, the little boy, was in for his twelve-month checkup. His mother told me this would be the last time I would see Randy as the biological father wanted Randy back. The family thought they had no option but to return Randy. I asked the family to let me think about it. Randy had been adopted when he was eighteen weeks old. He had been living with his biological father and his girlfriend prior to his being adopted. The father worked intermittently and social services said the condition of the house was deplorable. This alone would not be enough to prevent the father from getting Randy back. I reviewed Randy's previous medical records and plotted his height and weight on a growth chart. It was obvious that he had not grown well during his first eighteen weeks. After his adoption, his growth was very good. At eleven months his height and weight were at the fiftieth percentile and his development was now normal. Randy's chart also revealed several additional significant concerns about his development at the age when he was adopted. Randy lacked a social smile, could not raise his head when placed on his stomach, and had head lag when pulled up by his arms. A four-and-one-half month old infant should be able to do these things.

When the adoption hearing came, I provided this information to the court. The judge reviewed the social information, the growth information, and the development information. The judge ruled that

Randy would stay with his adoptive parents. The ruling was final. (It was later discovered that the natural paternal grandmother wanted the boy.)

Little Bobby

I gave a patient what would be his last physical exam. The young man was 6 feet 2 inches and 256 pounds and headed off to the University of Colorado to play football. His mom always referred to him as Little Bobby. All college football players are required to get a physical. So Little Bobby asked the CU football coach if he needed to have another physical exam as he had one with me. The coach asked Little Bobby what kind of doctor had done his physical. When Little Bobby said his pediatrician, all the coaches roared in laughter.

Adoptions

When I first entered practice in 1963, adoptions were very common. Some babies were adopted as soon as possible in as short as one to two months or as fast as an evaluation could be done. If the adoption was prearranged, the adoptive parents took the baby home from the hospital nursery.

In 1973, when the United States Supreme Court legalized abortion (Roe v. Wade), adoptions rapidly dried up. Adoption agencies turned to foreign countries for infants and children. The main sources of adoptive children were Eastern Europe and China. Later, some children were adopted from Central America. However, at some point, the State Department closed adoptions from Central America, and they may still be closed. Adoptions were halted because the origins of the babies were unknown and the adoptions were brokered by accountants who charged as much as thirty thousand dollars.

All adoptive children from foreign countries are screened for a number of infectious diseases such as hepatitis, tuberculosis, bacterial gastroenteritis, etc.

Typically, the Eastern European adoptive children had been very well cared for physically. However, they did not have significant human contact such as being held or rocked. As a result, when they came to the United States, it was very difficult for them to bond with their adoptive parents. These children also tended to be a little older, between two to four years old.

Chinese babies were not cared for physically, and some of them arrived with serious infections. On the other hand, these babies had a lot of human contact and bonded fairly easily. Almost invariably, all the adoptive children from China were girls. Although I once saw a baby boy adopted from China. Since this was nearly unheard of, I asked the parents how this was possible. The parents explained that his Chinese parents rejected him because he was born with an undescended testicle. Ironically, by the time I saw him, his testicle had descended.

One of the saddest adoption cases was a seven-year-old from India. He had not bonded with anyone. He was sent to an excellent child psychiatrist for evaluation. The mother called me the next day and said the psychiatrist said they should send him back to the adoption agency. I told her I thought this was very premature and we needed to give the situation more time. He also had a hole in between the two upper chambers of his heart (atrial septal defect) that required cardiac surgery. The surgery went well.

Unfortunately, it soon became apparent that the boy was physically abusive to the family's two biological children. He completely stopped communicating with the parents. Several large knives were missing from the kitchen. One night the parents woke and found him standing next to their bed with a large butcher knife. He was seen again by the child psychiatrist. There was an opening in a daytime psychiatric therapy center. The child psychiatrist felt that if the boy was treated for five or six years, that maybe things would get better. Because the family continued to fear for their lives, and their two biological children's safety, he was returned to the adoption agency. Despite the circumstances, the family felt a lot of guilt.

Faith

More recently there have been some open adoptions. An open adoption is where the mother of the baby meets the adoptive parents.

A staff member of our practice and her husband had tried to get pregnant for five years, including two in vitro procedures. Unfortunately, they could not conceive. Initially the husband was opposed to adoption but subsequently changed his mind.

Parents of a pregnant sixteen-year-old approached the couple and asked if they would like to adopt their daughter's baby. Their daughter was due to deliver in about three months and they wanted to choose the family. Again, the husband struggled with the idea of adoption but subsequently agreed. He reiterated they would only adopt a Caucasian baby as he did not want a biracial child. The young mother (girl) assured them this was not possible. The adoptive parents met the young girl and went to all her obstetrician (OB) appointments and attended the delivery. However, the daughter gave birth to a biracial baby. A social worker told the adopting couple they had twenty-four hours to decide whether they would go through with the adoption. The couple went through with the adoption and the child is her father's delight. He often came in with the child when she was sick and it was obvious that she was the apple of his eye.

Hidden agendas

Sometimes patients don't always tell you why they have made an appointment. So I walked into an examination room where a seventeen-year-old young lady was waiting. I asked, "How can I help you today?" She informed me that she'd had a bad cough for two days, but she had no fever or congestion and had been attending school. Her physical exam was normal. I suggested she try some over-the-counter cough medicine and started to leave. As I put my hand on the doorknob, she asked, "Can you get a venereal disease by having oral sex?" I sat back down and told her "Yes." After some discussion, I ordered appropriate lab tests. She said, "Thank you very much and please don't tell my mother." I can't remember how the tests turned out and I didn't tell the mother. However, the mother might have found out if she read her explanation of benefits (EOB) from her insurance company.

In a similar situation, the schedule said that Richard was here to get a sore throat and cough checked. He had no fever and his physical exam was completely normal. When he was getting ready to leave, he asked, "Could you check me for venereal disease?"

Electronic medical records (EMR)

Before I left practice, we switched to electronic medical records. Before long, I learned that there could be problems with this new technology.

My wife, Renee, had an eye infection, and she used some antibiotic eye drops we had at the house. But when her eye became very red and appeared more infected, a friend took her to the emergency room. When she returned, I asked her what the doctor had said. She told me that the CT scan showed that she did not have orbital cellulites. I said, "Good, but what did the doctor find when he examined you?" Much to my surprise, she said, "He didn't examine me." "He didn't check your eyes, ears, and throat? He didn't listen to your heart and lungs?" I asked. She answered, "No, he didn't do any of that... but he did give me a prescription for some antibiotic eye drops."

The next morning she was worse. She went to see her ophthalmologist. The ophthalmologist determined that the ER doctor prescribed the same family of antibiotic eye drops that my wife had used before going to the ER. He said she was obviously having an allergic reaction to those drops. A change in medication cleared the infection in several days.

Because her treatment at the emergency room concerned me, I requested her medical records. The records indicated that the doctor had done a complete physical exam and a complete neurological exam. I later learned that with electronic medical records, a doctor can document a complete physical exam or neurological exam with one mouse click. I filed complaints with the hospital, the medical board, and the doctor's malpractice insurance carrier. Since no one ever responded, I don't know the results of these complaints. I do know that this doctor still practices at the same hospital.

Coincidentally, this same doctor saw two of my patients over the next several months. One had a concussion and the other had a seizure. Similar to my wife, they both got CT scans of the head that were normal. My examinations and discussions with both patients also revealed this doctor again failed to perform physical and neurological exams. I discovered their concussions when I conducted my own neurological examinations. When starting the exam, I thought, this should go quickly since they both had this examination by the ER doctor. Not unsurprisingly, they both responded identically: "The doctor did not give me a neurological exam."

One of the problems with electronic medical records is that they allow doctors, like this ER doctor, to effortlessly and inaccurately document exams or treatments that were never provided. This creates a false documentation, and any dispute will be the doctor's word (backed up by the falsified records) versus the patient's word. Similarly, a hospital physician can copy his rounding notes from the previous day, make a few changes, and paste them into the rounding notes for the current day or any day.

Ice skater

A mother and daughter rented an apartment in Denver. The pediatrician father and the rest of the family stayed in Tulsa. The daughter had come to Denver to train under Carlo Fassi, the world-renowned ice skating coach. Because Denver was a temporary home, I only saw her for illnesses and injuries. Several years later I was watching the Winter Olympics, and I recognized the daughter when she was on the podium receiving a bronze medal.

Molly

Molly came in for her nine-month physical. It was concerning that she was not verbalizing. This was at a time when hearing was not checked in the newborn nursery. Shortly after her birth, a relative who was an internationally known audiologist had seen her socially and had not noticed anything abnormal. Molly's hearing was checked during my evaluation and she was found to be totally deaf. An audiologist at Porter Hospital, Doreen Pollock, was able to teach Molly to speak. Molly's speech was so good that she was selected to read the Christmas Story at her school. No one in the audience could tell that she was deaf.

Ballet Dancer

Every time I saw Jennifer for her annual checkup she was taking ballet lessons. I can't remember her exact age when she told me she had advanced into toe shoes. I kept up with her progress since she had a little sister that was still attending our practice. Shortly after Jennifer finished high school, her mother told me Jennifer had tried out for a prestigious ballet school in New York City and had been accepted. Five years later, Jennifer came into the office with her little sister. She had decided to retire from ballet and attend college. She said she enjoyed the ballet, but it was very hard work and there was little time to do anything else.

Professional athletes

Parents, coaches, and friends often see a talented young athlete and believe he or she will get a college scholarship and might even be able to play professionally. However, the reality is that a very small number of youth athletes ever make it to the pros. According to James Michener's book *Sports in America*, only about twenty-five college athletes make a professional basketball team. Only three hundred thirty-three make a professional football team. Baseball is somewhere in between those numbers. The cut down from high school football to college football is similarly drastic. About one million young men play football in high school, but only twenty-five thousand play college football.

Not only is the reality of the numbers stark, but other factors can conspire against athletes talented enough to make the pros. Years ago I had a patient named Sammy who played football for the University of Texas and then for Wyoming. He then tried out for the Minnesota Vikings as an undrafted free agent. Even though he was small for a defensive back, the starting defensive backs felt he was better than they were. However, the Vikings cut him and kept the veterans because they were owed guaranteed money. Sammy was not only a very good player but extremely knowledgeable. He later became the receivers coach at the Air Force Academy and later the offensive coordinator at the Naval Academy.

Another family under my care had three sons and one daughter. They were all excellent athletes. The boys played football and baseball. One of the boys held the Colorado State Football rushing record for many years. One college offered him both a football and baseball scholarship. However, a $1.8 million signing bonus with a major league team was too much to turn down. During his 13 years in the majors, he was a solid player, but not a great player. His older brother played a few years in the National League and then a number of years in the Cuban league.

During a checkup during his senior year, I asked a patient named Kevin who was the better baseball player, him or his brother? Without hesitation, Kevin said he was the better player. He played at Louisiana State University for four years, during which time they won the National Championship. Apparently, he was right because he was drafted into the majors as a pitcher and still pitches to this day.

Steve was 6 feet 4 inches and 230 pounds and played quarterback for the Denver Broncos. His daughter was in the hospital, and blood samples were needed from both he and his wife to help with the diagnosis. In the early 1960s, the Broncos were terrible. On the day before his daughter was hospitalized, Steve was sacked 13 times. The next day at the hospital, he was so sore he could not raise his arms to get into a gown. When the nurse came to draw his blood, he said that he just could not do that as it would be too painful.

Christian McCaffrey and his brothers were patients of mine. Like their parents, these young men were outstanding athletes. McCaffrey set the Colorado High School record of 141 touchdowns. He also set the record for all-purpose yards at 8,845 yards. In 2015 at Stanford, he set a record of 3,814 all-purpose yards and broke Barry

Sanders's record. In the Rose Bowl defeat of Iowa, he had 361 all-purpose yards (a Rose Bowl record). Many thought he should have won the Heisman Trophy award, but he finished second. Christian was drafted eighth in the NFL by the Carolina Panthers. He also has been all pro and was at one time the highest-paid running back in NFL history. Christian is the third player in NFL history to rush over 1,000 yards and have over 1,000 receiving yards in a single season. Currently, McCaffrey plays for the San Francisco 49ers.

Cunningham

A nineteen-year-old brought in her one-year-old baby sister for a checkup. She explained to me that her mother had died and her father recently married a woman who had never been around young children and could not raise the baby. The father asked his daughter if she would raise the child. The daughter agreed to adopt the child. (The daughter was the oldest of six siblings and had been around children for many years.)

Over the years I would ask the mother/sister if she had told her daughter/sister the true relationship, and she always answered "Not yet." One day, when the adopted girl turned thirteen, she found her original birth certificate. She asked, "Who is this person who has the same first and middle name as I do and the same birthday?" Her mother/sister then finally told the girl that her grandfather was actually her father and she was actually her older sister. After hearing the truth, the teenage girl was very upset and required a significant amount of counseling to help her deal with this difficult reality.

The teenage years can be very difficult, and withholding this news made them more challenging for this young girl. To avoid this type of scenario, and for many other reasons, adoptive parents should let the adopted child know that they have been adopted from day one. The adopted child should not be able to remember a time when they did not know they were adopted.

ALMOST FIFTY YEARS' EXPERIENCE AS A PEDIATRICIAN

Patients become doctors

Over the years a number of my patients became physicians. Since these young adults had outgrown my care, I would only learn about it from a younger sibling who was still coming to see me. Sometimes the mother would call me to tell me that their child had just graduated from medical school. On several occasions, a young person would come up to me and introduce themselves. "Do you remember me? I was your patient, and now I am in medical school." Regardless of how I heard, I was always gratified to hear this news.

Andrew

Andrew was born into a poor black family in Washington, DC, and was one of eight children. Andrew met a family from Denver that worked with the federal government and spent a lot of time in Washington. The Denver family befriended Andrew over time when he did small jobs for them. When he was about eight years old, they invited him to spend the summer in Denver. The family told Andrew that he should write a letter to his mother. But when they gave him paper and pencil, Andrew could not write. Andrew had severe learning disabilities. From that summer on, he lived with the Denver family and they got him into special education classes.

Andrew went to Cherry Creek High School (CCHS) his sophomore year. He was a very good football player, and he continued to get extra help in the classroom. After our usual loss in the playoffs, we were at a bar, and Coach Tesone said the family was moving back to Washington. The father was an administrative aide to Senator Armstrong. Andrew needed a place to live his senior year. Since our son Jon was a senior and played football, we volunteered.

Andrew was the first and only person in his family to graduate from high school. He went to Mesa College in Grand Junction, Colorado, on a football scholarship. He still needed extra help in the classroom. A coach recognized this early on as he had a son with learning problems. Coach directed Andrew to the right classes and resources.

We saw Andrew several times over the years. We received a call one spring from Andrew, he was in town and wanted to take us to dinner. Andrew is married and has two sons and two grandchildren. He is a deacon in his church and started a successful moving company. Just before she died, his mother told him that he was born in prison. I often wondered if his mother had been in prison for drugs and if this was the cause of his learning disabilities. Andrew told us that the CCHS football program played a huge role in his success in life. The many lessons he learned playing CCHS football had served him well. What a success story!

Multiple sclerosis

One does not usually think that multiple sclerosis (MS) is a pediatric disease. However, several cases come to mind. Josh was a junior in high school when he was diagnosed with MS. There are several types of MS and Josh's was unrelenting and progressive. Despite this, Josh finished college and went to medical school. However, his MS made it obvious that he would not be able to practice most specialties. Josh became a psychiatrist and counseled people with disabilities. He died far too young in his early thirties.

Jennifer was a very talented violinist. She earned a scholarship to a prominent music school in Texas. In her second year of music school, she was diagnosed with MS. Before long, she could no longer play the violin. Since then she has had multiple psychiatric issues.

William was diagnosed with MS his senior year in high school. His first symptoms were visual, and the ophthalmologist diagnosed him as having MS. William had relapsing-remitting MS. This type of MS is characterized by repeated attacks with periods of partial or complete recovery. William worked hard to maintain good health by eating well and exercising. He continues to have intermittent attacks of MS.

"Why am I so short?"

At his nineteen-year checkup, Joel was four feet eleven inches. X-rays showed his growth centers were closed. As a child, he had bad asthma, and his mother said the medicine she got from Mexico helped him a lot. I explained to her that it was probably a steroid that could close his growth centers. Since it helped his asthma, she was not interested in stopping the medication. Unfortunately, it was determined it was a steroid and had permanently closed his growth centers. Since his growth centers were closed, growth hormones would not help. Joel's adult height would always be four feet eleven inches.

Assumption

When a parent brought in several children, we assumed they all had the same thing. The mother said the children had a fever, sore throat, cough, and stomach pain. The first child had mainly a sore throat, and his strep test was positive. The second child had a bad cough with a fever, and his influenza test was positive. The third child had no cough or sore throat but bad stomach pain. He had his appendix out later that day.

Short, short stories

The price is right? In 1963, a diphtheria, pertussis, tetanus immunization (DPT) shot was $3. Even though a much safer DPT vaccine was developed, the legal aspects raised the price to over $30.

EpiPens. An EpiPen is a prefilled syringe with epinephrine to be given for severe allergic reactions. The amount of epinephrine in the syringes is probably less than $1. At one point the price was raised to $135 and later to over $600. These pens must be refilled every year. In 49 years of practice, I never had a patient use their EpiPen for an allergic reaction.

PE tubes (pressure equalizing tubes). These tubes were placed through the eardrum for children having chronic ear infections. It was felt this fluid decreased hearing and interfered with speech development. Jack L. Paradise, MD, a renowned otolaryngologist, showed that speech development was not affected by the fluid in the ear.

Once Dr. Paradise revealed this information, the number of PE tube procedures was greatly reduced.

Gastroesophageal reflux (GERD). Almost all newborns spit up, but by one year of age, almost none continue to spit up. If the child was not gaining weight, a Nissen procedure was performed. This tightens the esophageal sphincter. A Denver pediatric surgeon performed this procedure in over 900 healthy, growing, well babies simply because the spitting up was inconvenient for the parents. This is malpractice.

Teething. Teething gets blamed for a lot of things. Studies have shown that fever, if any, is insignificant. If the baby has a significant fever, the baby needs to be evaluated for a serious illness such as meningitis, pneumonia, etc. If a teething baby is found to have an ear infection or gastroenteritis, this is a coincidence.

Visiting hours. Prior to the introduction of penicillin, children with strep infections were placed in a ward until their culture became negative. Parents were allowed to see the child two times per week through a glass window. Penicillin allowed parents to visit more frequently. Today, visiting hours are unrestricted, and parents are encouraged to stay with their child at all times. Sleeping chairs are provided for parents.

Participation. When I first went into practice, we made house calls. There were no emergency room (ER) doctors in the hospital to care for patients who went to the ER. In addition, there were no neonatal nurses to attend high-risk deliveries. These situations required the on-call physician from our practice to go to the ER to attend to our patient. Likewise, if a high-risk mother was going to deliver one of our patients, we had to attend the delivery. When your pager gave a signal, you needed to call in to get a message as no other details were provided.

Food allergies. For years, the conventional wisdom was to recommend that potential allergen foods not be introduced until a year after birth. Common allergen foods included items such as peanuts, eggs, milk, tree nuts, wheat, shellfish, fish, and soy. This was a mistake! It was later found that if these foods were introduced in small quantities prior to six months of age, a child would be much less likely to develop an allergy to a specific food. Guidelines now stress these foods should be introduced between four to six months of age when solid foods are introduced. SpoonfulONE™ contains all these foods. It comes in a powder to add to solids the child eats.

Unnecessary radiation. Most X-rays and CT scans are not required for a child with a headache, head trauma, or possible concussion. A thorough history and physical examination would eliminate the need for most of these studies.

Down syndrome. Many, many years ago, children born with Down syndrome were whisked away to institutions for the mentally retarded. Dr. Lula Lubchenco was a pediatrician and pioneer in the specialty of neonatology at Colorado General Hospital. Dr. Lubchenco was one of a number of parents who chose to take her Down syndrome child home. These children were loveable, and their development was much better with their families. They were able to perform basic tasks of self-care and even employment.

Umbilical hernias. In the past, umbilical hernias were repaired by two years of age. Later it was found that some of these hernias closed on their own as late as five years of age. It is now recommended to wait until age five to repair.

Bed rest. Bed rest was prescribed for children with acute rheumatic fever. A study using pedometers found that children put on bed rest were just as active as children not prescribed bed rest.

Aspirin and Reye's syndrome. Aspirin is no longer advised be given to very young children as it may cause Reye's syndrome. I once had a patient whose mother called and said her son was extremely restless and febrile. Before I left for hospital rounds that morning, I called the mother, who said the child had calmed down and was sleeping. Immediately I went to the child's home, and he was semicomatose. We went to Children's Hospital Colorado, and he was diagnosed with Reye's syndrome. Fortunately, this child made a full recovery.

Stomach ulcers. Stomach ulcers that run in families were once believed to be inherited, psychological, and a stress-induced condition. However, it was found that ulcers are caused by a bacterium called *Helicobacter pylori* (H. pylori). Treatment is with antibiotics.

Insurance companies leave doctors holding the bag! Families aren't the only ones who struggle with insurance companies. Insurance companies have become anything but traditional with their constant pressure to save money. Reimbursement was becoming more of a challenge for the physician. The insurance company's answer was for doctors to see more patients to make up for the deficit in income. One of the more innovative ways for one particular insurance carrier was to penalize the physician by taking the cost of lab work, X-rays, etc., out of the doctor's reimbursement. This extremely challenged a physician's decision making and process to treat patients. These insurance companies are no longer in business.

What's best for my child? Parents would often ask me what they could do to help their child's development. There is an excellent book by Burton L. White, *The First Three Years of Life*. In his book, White stressed that what parents do in the first three years of life determines how well a child develops. I encourage you to read White's findings.

Later, other studies provided crucial evidence to make a significant impact in a child's life and to maximize a child's language development: Starting at birth, they should hear thirty thousand words a day (yes, we do talk that much). This is extremely valuable! These thirty thousand words should come from parents, family members, and caregivers. What a child hears on television, iPads, telephones, and/or electronic devices does not count. Simply put, unplug! Talk to your child when you are at home, while taking walks, and while you're driving. This investment in your child is worth more than gold!

Other important pointers I give parents include always responding to infants. This creates better self-esteem. Share discoveries. Read to your child.

COMMENTS AND OBSERVATIONS BY PATIENTS AND PARENTS

- "My child's temperature is 103." The nurse asked the mother how she was taking it. "Pretty well under the circumstances," the mother responded.
- A mother who had recently moved to the U.S. from China called and said I needed to see her daughter right away as she was having a "severe immigrant headache."
- The same mother said she was checking her son's "auxiliary temperature" and that he was behind on his "enemazations."
- The sixth-grader told me he was glad that he got check marks on his report card as his parents did not know what they meant.

CHAPTER 7

Vaccines

Many say that vaccines were the most important public health advancement in the twentieth century. In his book, *Deadliest Enemy: Our War Against Killer Germs*, Michael T. Osterholm, PhD, MPH, states, "The biggest bang for the buck is vaccines." He quotes Seth Berkeley, MD, "Vaccines are among the most successful and cost-effective health investments in history." In addition, improved sanitation and antibiotics played a significant role in the decrease in mortality we saw before the twentieth century. It is also important to note that the incidence of infectious diseases had started to decline before the widespread use of vaccines. Cleaner water, sanitation, and the development of state health departments contributed to this improvement.

The smallpox vaccine was developed in 1797 by Edward Jenner. Jenner inoculated healthy individuals against smallpox by using the cowpox virus. The cowpox was put on scraped skin of the recipient. Persons inoculated in this manner were then protected against smallpox.

The late nineteenth century saw the development of many additional vaccines: cholera (1879), rabies (1885), tetanus (1890), typhoid fever (1896), and bubonic plague (1897) were developed.

The development of vaccines accelerated in the twentieth century. The list includes the following: tuberculosis (1921), diphtheria (1923), typhus (1937), influenza (1945), pertussis (whooping cough)

(1926), polio-Salk (1952), polio-Sabin (1962), measles (1963), mumps (1967), rubella (1970), chickenpox (1974), pneumococcal disease (1977), meningitis (1978), hepatitis B (1981), *Haemophilus influenzae* type B (HiB, 1985), hepatitis A (1992), Lyme disease (1998), and rotavirus (1998).

Twenty-first century vaccines includes the following: nasal influenza vaccine (2003), human papillomavirus (HPV, 2006), quadrivalent influenza vaccine (2012), enterovirus (2013), malaria (2015), Ebola (2015), COVID-19 (2020).

The COVID-19 vaccine was the fastest vaccine ever developed. In May of 2020, President Trump announced Operation Warp Speed (public and private partnership) to develop a vaccine against COVID-19. They were developed by the end of 2020 (in approximately nine months). By contrast, prior to the COVID-19 vaccine, mumps was the fastest developed vaccine. It took five years!

With respect to many illnesses that vaccines were developed for, many parents ask, "Aren't those just childhood diseases that every child gets?" In the United States, polio was nonexistent because of vaccinations until a recent isolated one-off case was reported in 2022. The smallpox vaccination has eliminated smallpox from the planet. For this reason, all remaining smallpox vaccines were going to be destroyed. However, this did not happen because both the United States and Russia still have the smallpox virus in their labs. This would allow additional vaccines to be made if needed, although both countries maintain stockpiles of smallpox vaccine.

Many of the diseases for which vaccines were produced can cause serious complications including death. A simple summary may be helpful:

Polio can cause paralysis, respiratory problems, and death.
Mumps can cause sterility and pancreatitis.
Pneumococcal can cause meningitis, pneumonia, and soft tissue infections.
Rotavirus can cause dehydration, hepatitis B, liver failure and liver cancer, and death.
Human papillomavirus (HPV) can cause cervical cancer.

Rabies almost always results in death.

Chickenpox causes severe secondary skin infections usually caused by streptococcus.

Tuberculosis causes severe lung disease, pneumonia, and death.

Rubella (German measles) affected twenty thousand infants between 1964 to 1965. Many of these babies were left deaf, blind, mentally retarded, and/or had cardiac defects. Measles can also cause mental retardation, hearing loss, and death. If a mother develops rubella during the late first trimester of her pregnancy, rubella may cause severe congenital heart disease, blindness, deafness, and/or death for the fetus.

Vaccines were made to prevent these severe complications. Other than whooping cough, many physicians have not seen most of these diseases for which vaccines were developed.

Before the development of vaccines, the impact of many of these illnesses were devastating. Prior to a vaccine, pertussis (whooping cough) reported 150,000 to 260,000 cases per year in the United States with 9,000 deaths. The coughing spells would last for weeks and the child had difficulty eating and drinking. Depending on how often and to the extent they became dehydrated, infants developed pneumonia, brain damage, seizures, retardation, and frequently died.

In 1952, before the Salk vaccine, there were 58,000 cases of polio reported in America. Polio affected mainly children, leaving many of them in braces or on crutches. There were 3 million cases annually with an average of 6,000 deaths per year.

Bacterial meningitis caused by *Haemophilus influenzae* type b (Hib) was the most common form of meningitis. Pneumococcal also caused numerous cases of bacterial meningitis. Approximately 600 children die each year from bacterial meningitis.

Given the progress made with vaccines, most think the era of pandemics is over. However, as recently proved by COVID-19, a new pandemic can occur at any time if a disease occurs for which there is no vaccine. Examples of pandemics include tuberculosis, cholera, bubonic plague, influenza, human immunodeficiency virus (HIV), acquired immunodeficiency syndrome (AIDS), typhus, and measles. History is marked by many notable and significant pandemics.

The Native American Pandemic (1500–1700). Previous to the arrival of European settlers, Native Americans had no contact with smallpox, measles, and influenza. These three diseases killed up to seventy percent (70 percent) of some tribes. Total deaths were estimated to be 1.5 million people.

Spanish flu (1918–1919): The death toll was 50–100 million men, women, and children. Other influenza pandemics include the Asian flu between 1856 to 1858, and a second pandemic of Asian flu between 1956 to 1958.

Human immunodeficiency virus (HIV, 1981 to present time). According to the latest statistics from HIV.gov, about 32.7 million people have died and 38.4 million people worldwide are infected. The number of deaths worldwide has steadily decreased from a high of over 2 million in 2004 to around 650,000. In the United States, there are about 34,000 to 37,000 new cases per year, but the number is dropping.

Worldwide, there are about 1.5 million newly diagnosed cases of acquired immunodeficiency syndrome (AIDS) per year, and some people don't even know they have it. Antiretroviral therapies have been very effective in combating AIDS. These therapies have resulted in an approximate 60 percent drop in HIV-related deaths since the peak of the pandemic in 2004. Prevention has been important in decreasing the number of new cases as well, because there is no AIDS vaccine and the virus is constantly mutating. HIV/AIDS is one of the most highly funded research projects by the National Institute of Health. However, some worry that funds have been and will continue to be diverted from AIDS research to COVID-19.

The black death (bubonic plague, 1335–1351). The plague disease, caused by the bacterium *Yersinia pestis*, is enzootic (commonly present) in populations of fleas carried by ground rodents.

Rats spread the disease along trade routes. The black death was the most devastating pandemic of all time, killing an estimated 75–200 million people. The black death is estimated to have killed 30 percent–60 percent of the European population. Historians estimate that it took over two hundred years for the world to regain the population lost to the black death.

The third bubonic plague (1835). This plague originated in China and spread throughout the world. For the next twenty years, it was spread to port cities. The total death toll was ten million.

Cholera. Before the purification of water, there were seven major pandemics in the last two hundred years. These infections were caused by a bacterium, *vibrio cholerae*. Some of these cholera pandemics caused hundreds of thousands of deaths. A Spanish physician, Jaime Ferrán, created a mass vaccine in 1885.

Typhus (1918, World War I). Some estimates assert that as many as eight million German soldiers died of typhus. Typhus was also a common cause of death in concentration camps.

Tuberculosis (TB). Caused by mycobacterium, TB has consistently been the leading infectious cause of death in the world. For this reason, and because it has been around for thousands of years, TB is often referred to as the forgotten pandemic. The World Health Organization (WHO) estimates that 1.8 billion, or 25 percent, of the world's population are infected with TB, including latent TB, which is not transmissible. In 2018, around 10 million people became ill from TB with 1.5 million deaths. This bacterial infection is spread through the air and is treatable with antibiotics. However, resistance to TB antibiotics is becoming a problem. HIV and TB are a deadly combination. HIV weakens the immune system making TB infection more likely. The death rate for TB is around 45 percent, but that death rate increases to nearly 100 percent for HIV-positive individuals.

Will we see pandemics in the future? The smallpox virus currently only exists in two labs in the world (Russia and the United States). The bubonic plague, typhus, and cholera are all treatable with antibiotics and fluids. During any given year, influenza can infect approximately 35 million Americans, with annual deaths estimated from 12,000 to over 50,000. The Centers for Disease Control (CDC) estimates that there are 250,000–650,000 deaths from influenza in the world each year.

Many diseases for which vaccines have been developed do not change or mutate significantly. Therefore, the vaccines do not need to be constantly changed. However, the influenza vaccine must be modified annually. The pharmaceutical industry continually develops antiviral drugs and some have been effective against influenza. But these antivirals must be started within 24 to 48 hours after the onset of symptoms. Influenza is a leading candidate to cause a pandemic because of its constantly mutating nature. Because of its ability to mutate, the possibility exists that an influenza strain could develop that current vaccines would be ineffective against and that is also resistant to current antiviral medications.

As of September 2022, COVID-19 is now present in all continents, even Antarctica. More importantly, worldwide governmental responses shelled out a profound shock to all aspects of human life. Just about every facet of life was impacted, including stock markets, almost all businesses, schools, and travel.

Unfortunately, many vaccines are viewed as harmful. The Internet is full of negative information about vaccines despite significant efforts to censor such content. Apparently, most people who feel positive about vaccines tend not to post on the Internet. In his 2007 book *Vaccine: The Controversial Story of Medicine's Greatest Lifesaver*, Arthur Allen discusses that historically, at one time or another, controversy has accompanied the development of almost all vaccines.

Autism and the Vaccine Myth

A recent and unfortunate major vaccine controversy is the claim that the measles, mumps, rubella (MMR) vaccine causes autism. This controversy was initiated by a 1998 study published in *The Lancet* (a highly respected British medical journal). The study's author, Andrew Wakefield, presented a mere twelve cases with no control group. Based on this small study, he proposed that there was a link between the MMR vaccine and autism. The study received wide publicity. Some incorrectly concluded that a link had been established between the MMR vaccine and autism. While both the MMR vaccination and autism occur in early childhood, this temporal coincidence does not mean that autism was caused by the MMR vaccination, nor did the study establish a causal link. Epidemiological studies were subsequently conducted and published refuting the association. A preservative, thimerosal, was thought by some to be the cause of autism. Thimerosal has been removed from most vaccines with the exception of one flu vaccine, and there has been no decrease in autism.

Antivaccine advocates (antivaxxers) immediately started using Wakefield's study as proof that vaccines cause autism. Wakefield's study was the subject of a feature on television investigative series *60 Minutes*. Jenny McCarthy—fashion model, 1994 Playmate of the Year, actress, TV celebrity, and porn star—was an avid antivaccine spokesperson and became the face of the antivaxx movement. McCarthy would regularly state that her son developed autism after receiving the MMR vaccine and she claims that she cured his autism. McCarthy's cure included speech therapy, special diets, and other suggestions from the Internet.

Twenty-four years after the Wakefield study was published, the claim that MMR causes autism still persists. These claims persist despite the fact that the Wakefield study has been completely discredited. The well-known investigative journalist, Brian Deer, revealed in a series of articles that shed a spotlight on Wakefield findings. Deer reported that Wakefield had serious and undisclosed conflicts of interest and manipulated the data, and that the study was essentially an elaborate fraud. In 2004, *The Lancet* published a brief retraction of the study. The retraction did state that the data did not support the claim that MMR causes autism. The retraction was signed by ten of the thirteen original study authors. In 2010 (twelve years after the original study was published), *The Lancet* again completely retracted the original article proposing a link between MMR and autism. Wakefield was called an ethical cheat who falsified data. As Brian Deer discovered, Wakefield also had received money from attorneys representing antivaccine parents. Dr. Andrew Wakefield lost his medical credentials in 2010. Despite the overwhelming evidence to the contrary, Wakefield still maintains that MMR causes autism.

One more study is not going to change the opinions of antivaccine advocates. However, a study done in Denmark was reported in 2019 in the *Journal of Internal Medicine*. The authors looked at 657,461 children who had received the MMR vaccine. Of those,

ALMOST FIFTY YEARS' EXPERIENCE AS A PEDIATRICIAN

6,517 children were diagnosed with autism. That's 0.0099 percent! Dr. Anders Hviid, the lead author of the article, stressed that measles disease was much greater of a risk than the MMR vaccine. I agree that the vaccine is a much lower risk than the disease. For this reason, all seven of my children, eighteen grandchildren, and four great-grandchildren have been vaccinated.

COMMENTS AND OBSERVATIONS BY PATIENTS AND PARENTS

- A mother asked me if I could call in a prescription to Walgreens at southeast plasma.
- The mother said her baby had diarrhea. When I asked what it looked like, she said, "Cheddar cheese." (Tschetter, the author's last name, is pronounced "cheddar.")
- A patient asked if I would use "biodegradable stitches" as he did not want to come in to get his stitches out.

CHAPTER 8

Mary Ann
A Grandfather's Perspective of a Tragedy

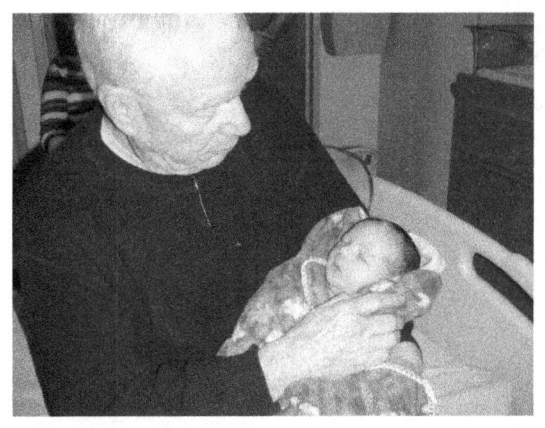

The author with his granddaughter, Maryann

Introduction

The story of Mary Ann's death is about one of the most difficult times of my life and that of my family. This tragedy was even more painful than the agonizing malignant brain tumor suffered by my grandson Zach and the premature birth of my grandson James.

Out of respect for our son and daughter-in-law, they will remain nameless. Pronouns such as son, daughter-in-law, mother, father, wife, parents, and couple will be used to refer to Mary Ann's parents.

In the fall of 2005, our son called and told us he and his wife were expecting a baby girl and she would be born in 2006. Shortly after, the couple moved from California to Olympia, Washington, because our son had taken a job with the Salvation Army. My wife, Renee, and I went to Olympia in October to celebrate the second birthday of their first son. During the visit, our daughter-in-law informed us that in the State of Washington, hospitals and physicians did not allow vaginal births after a mother has had a caesarean delivery (C-section). Vaginal birth after C-section is commonly referred to as VBAC. The birth of their first child had been by C-section due to our daughter-in-law's high blood pressure.

A home VBAC delivery was planned.

The Fateful Meeting of Pam Golliet

Unfortunately, our son and daughter-in-law met Pam Golliet (hereafter referred to as Golliet) at an Integrated Community Alternatives Network (ICAN) meeting in October 2005. They discussed with Golliet their desire to have an at-home VBAC. Golliet assured them that she had done many VBACs with patients at home. Golliet also assured our daughter-in-law that if at any time she requested to go to the hospital, she would be taken immediately and a C-section would be performed.

Based on Golliet's representations at the initial meeting, our son and his wife met with her again to discuss an at-home VBAC. Golliet lied to them when she told them that she had been doing VBACs for years (implied twenty years). We later learned from her own website that during that time, Golliet had primarily practiced childbirth education, been a doula, and was a board-certified doula (support person for laboring mothers) and lactation consultant. We also later learned from Golliet's website that she had only received her midwifery license in February of 2005. Therefore, she had been doing home deliveries for less than a year when she delivered Mary Ann. Despite this, Golliet told our son and daughter-in-law that she had attended over 250 births and delivered over 100 babies. Such statements were extremely misleading. Golliet never made it clear that nearly all the births she had attended were as a doula in addition to other flat-out lies. Example of one lie: How could she possibly have delivered over 11 babies per month in the 9-month period between February 2005 when she became licensed and October 2005 (when she met with these parents)? Golliet's website did not mention whether any of the babies she delivered were VBACs.

On Golliet's website, she also boldly bragged that "someone had to do at-home VBACs" even though her malpractice insurance did not provide coverage for home VBACs. Golliet reiterated this in the media. She basically stated something to the effect that, "Even though I know my medical malpractice insurance will not cover me, someone has to do at-home VBACs. My medical malpractice insurance expressly said they specifically excluded at-home VBACs and will not cover at-home VBACs." How brazen! Golliet knew that her medical malpractice insurance company would not cover liability for at-home VBACs. She knowingly defied her medical malpractice carrier by doing at-home VBACs. "I'm taking a risk," she arrogantly stated. Unfortunately, it was this young couple that took the risk that ended in tragedy. Despite all her bravado, Golliet notified the insurance carrier the day after Mary Ann's death and made changes to her website that same day as well.

The prenatal visits

After the initial meeting, our daughter-in-law had three or four prenatal visits with Golliet. At no time did Golliet perform a pelvic exam or an ultrasound, even though mother requested an ultrasound to check the baby's position and general growth. A pelvic exam may or may not have revealed that Mary Ann was in a breach position. However, an ultrasound would have revealed this for sure! Golliet told our daughter-in-law that ultrasounds were unreliable this far into her pregnancy. Furthermore, she said that all important information could be determined through the fetal scope and an external examination of the womb. During the prenatal visits, Golliet continued to reinforce the parents' impression that she had done many at-home VBACs.

Although she never conducted an ultrasound, in January of 2006, Golliet referred our daughter-in-law to a chiropractor because she knew the position of the baby was breech. Both our son and daughter-in-law were skeptical about going to a chiropractor. However, Golliet told them that the chiropractor would perform a Webster procedure to switch the baby into a normal birth position. While skeptical, our daughter-in-law finally went to the chiropractor who performed the Webster procedure.

The labor and delivery

My wife, Renee, had gone to Olympia, Washington, in anticipation of Mary Ann's birth and to assist watching our grandson. At some point, Renee let me know that our daughter-in-law was going into labor. I called Golliet from my office in Denver and said, "Take care of mother and the baby." Golliet said, "I will." Renee specifically asked Golliet during this time if the baby was in a breech position. Golliet reassured Renee that the baby was not in a breech position and that the baby was head down. Golliet's reassurances were based on nothing, because Golliet had absolutely no factual or medical basis to make such reassurances.

After several episodes of false labor, mother was unquestionably in labor. Golliet was notified and returned to deliver the baby. Upon arrival, Golliet performed the only pelvic exam during labor and said that she could feel the baby's head and hair. Our daughter-in-law said she was in extreme pain and asked if they shouldn't go to the hospital. Golliet said that they should wait a while and see what happens. Golliet never mentioned going to the hospital again. Golliet said the baby's hand was by her face and that was the cause of the pain the mother was having and that the labor was progressing nicely.

Our daughter-in-law asked if she could have her blood pressure checked again as it was high when Golliet first arrived. She was concerned because she had experienced high blood pressure when she delivered her first child. Golliet told her that it wasn't necessary. Our daughter-in-law continued to be worried and asked if she should have another pelvic exam. Again, Golliet said that it wasn't necessary. Golliet told our daughter-in-law that she could tell by "other factors" how far along she was in labor.

Golliet then asked the father if he wanted to feel the head and hair. Our son did feel the baby and said, "That can't be the head... it's the buttocks." Golliet responded by saying that the head gets squeezed in labor and therefore feels mushy. At this point, anyone with any experience would have realized that the baby was breech. However, it took Golliet a few minutes more to realize the baby was breech. She ordered mother to push harder. Mary Ann's heartbeat dropped. Mother frantically requested to call 911, but Golliet ignored her. Golliet was reaching inside and pulling the baby. Golliet delivered the baby's body but could not deliver the head for another five minutes. The doula at the delivery called 911 on her own, during which time Mary Ann was born.

Mary Ann had a pulse. Minimal respiratory efforts by the baby were observed. Golliet had a simple rubber bulb syringe to suck out the baby's nose and mouth. Golliet did not have adequate equipment to care for an infant in such a severe state. She should have had the equipment to intubate and breathe for the baby. When the paramedics arrived, Golliet said that she had a "surprise breech" and abruptly left. The baby was readied for transport. When the paramedics saw all the blood mother had lost, they said she also should be transported to Providence St. Peter Hospital.

After the ambulance left, I called Golliet from Denver. I could not restrain my anger, "You killed our baby! You had twenty-four hours to figure out what position the baby was in." She arrogantly responded that she had been up for twenty-four hours, was very tired, and needed to go home to get some sleep.

Details from the delivery

A statement made by the doula, Cook, who attended the delivery stated in her deposition that "everything was in chaos!". Additional excerpts from her statement are as follows:

PAUL N. TSCHETTER, MD

Jan. 17, 2006

    Pam [Golliet] called to say that mother's blood pressure was elevated and probably would be going to the hospital.
    I arrived. Fetal heart tones were checked every hour to half hour during labor. Mother had one vaginal exam that I was aware of that morning. She [Pam Golliet] stated to me that she would only do them if necessary for information.
    Fetal heart tones are being checked every 15 minutes. They are strong and consistent.
    Mother is asking for pain relief and Pam gave her Arnica. During the next hour, Pam [Golliet] discussed alternatives to pain coping and transferring to hospital for birth with both parents. Mother appeared upset and concerned about the time frame that it was taking to have her baby. We continued to discuss the option of going to the hospital. Pam [Golliet] thought it might be time for pushing.

Jan. 18, 2006

    The baby's body was out; the umbilical chord [sic] was very pale. She (Pam Golliet) said the head was stuck and she could not deliver the head for five minutes. I asked her if she wanted me to call 911. I repeated the request two more times and then I told Pam (Golliet) I was going to call 911; she said, "yes, go call." I went to another room and called 911. As I ran back to where mother was, I saw that the baby had been delivered. I grabbed the O2 tank, *redacted* grabbed the stethescope [sic] and bulb syringe at Pam's request. I knelt down on the floor listened to the baby's HR (heart rate) while delivering blow by oxygen…until CPR was initiated. HR was around 40 bpm (beats per minute), I gave the stethescope [sic] to Pam and said we need to start CPR right now. There was no equipment to intubate Mary Ann.

When the paramedics arrived they took over and were unable to intubate the baby.

Summary of other crucial comments and observations made by Cook:

- "No Blood Pressures were taken while I was there, nor did I take any blood pressures."
- "I do not recall Pam [Golliet] ever talking about the need to take mother's blood pressure, although it was elevated that morning."
- "The midwife did one vaginal exam while I was there."
- "Pam [Golliet] did state that she had felt lots of hair on the baby during the one vaginal exam."
- "My understanding was that the baby was head down. She [Pam Golliet] was surprised to see no hair. The father did say…what he was seeing was not her [the baby's] head."
- "Mother requested transfer to the hospital. I was not present when mother talked with Pam about transferring. Mother and I talked about going to the hospital and not failing if she did so."
- "I know mother was very discouraged about making the choice to go. I tried to reinforce that she could go any time. I told her that I would go with her if she needed me there."
- "I initiated the request to call 911 with Pam."
- "While I had gone to call 911, I was not present at the time that the baby's head was delivered."
- "While I administered the breaths, Pam [Golliet] administered the compressions. The paramedics took over when they arrived."

Providence St. Peter Hospital

After arrival, Mary Ann was resuscitated and placed on a ventilator. She was not breathing on her own. Arrangements were made to transfer her to the Neonatal Intensive Care Unit (NICU) at Tacoma General Hospital. While waiting for Mary Ann to be transferred, her father baptized her in the name of the Father, and of the Son, and of the Holy Spirit.

Mother was taken to the operating room. The doctors also informed mother that she might need a hysterectomy and a blood transfusion. Unbelievably, Golliet had the nerve to stop by. Even more incredibly, she seemed angry and emphatically stated that mother would not need a hysterectomy or any blood and would be just fine.

Our son called me from the hospital. He had good news and bad news. The good news was that overall our daughter-in-law was okay, even though she had lost a lot of blood. The bad (tragic) news was that Mary Ann was in critical condition and not breathing on her own. I felt helpless because I was still in Denver seeing patients and my flight to Seattle was not until later that day. Words cannot relate how distressing our son's call was. I didn't know all the facts of the situation, but I knew enough as a doctor to be certain that Mary Ann was not going to survive. Despite this, I kept praying for her.

Tacoma General Hospital

Mary Ann was transferred to the NICU at Tacoma General. After being released, our daughter-in-law immediately took the approximate thirty-minute ride to Tacoma to see and hold Mary Ann for the first time. Mary Ann was on a ventilator and had intravenous (IV) lines. Mary Ann showed no response to stimuli. I can't remember why I felt some hope, but I do recall feeling slightly hopeful after the neurologist came by to evaluate Mary Ann. This was probably false hope on my part driven by the need just to feel some optimism. The doctors and nurses at Tacoma General were unbelievable. The neonatologists were with the same group that practices with some of the neonatologists in Denver. I was confident and grateful that Mary Ann was getting the best care.

A neonatologist informed our son and daughter-in-law after an electroencephalogram (EEG) that Mary Ann was brain dead. These young parents had to make the decision that no parent should ever have to make—whether or not to continue life support for a child. On the third day of Mary Ann's life, her parents together made the decision to discontinue life support. In the NICU, our son looked down at his daughter. Her eyes were closed, and the only sound was the ventilator pushing air into her limp body as he stroked her head.

After life support was discontinued, Mary Ann continued to breathe and had a strong heartbeat for six hours. Because of this, the brief possibility of Mary Ann living occurred to everyone. Her parents experienced unimaginable anguish. One moment they are holding their newborn child as she continued to breathe, knowing that it would stop at any second. But during this time they experienced a brief flash of horror that a severely neurologically damaged Mary Ann might live. From inevitable death to a life worse than death.

After approximately six hours, Mary Ann went to be with the Lord. The nurses then asked if we wanted to bathe Mary Ann. So her father and I did. The nurses also gave us a little white dress to put on her.

The funerals

A brief funeral for Mary Ann was held the next day in Olympia, Washington, at the Salvation Army Worship Center where her father worked. He got up and said a few words. Obviously still reeling from Mary Ann's death, it was difficult for our son and daughter-in-law to make any sense of what had transpired. Similarly, everyone present was experiencing difficulty in understanding those events. Arrangements were then made for Mary Ann to be transported back to Denver.

Two days later, Mary Ann's service was held in Denver at the Hampden Gardens Funeral Home. The entire family came early to view Mary Ann. She was beautiful and at peace. Father Tadeusz

Kopczynski, a Catholic priest from Poland, conducted the service. Because of his accent, one had to listen very carefully. Readings were assigned to Mary Ann's father and myself. I will always remember one poignant part of the service. Father Tadeusz said, "Mother and Father, always remember that you have two children. One is here, and one is in heaven." Also etched in my mind is our son carrying the tiny casket to the hearse at the conclusion of the service. Everyone went to the gravesite where Mary Ann was buried next to her great-grandmother and her step-great-grandfather.

Letter to Golliet

After the funeral, I wrote a letter to Golliet on January 27, 2006.

Ms. Golliet:

Following Mary Ann's delivery you went home very tired. "I've been up for 24 hours." Mary Ann's parents went home to an empty nursery. Her mother went home with full breasts and no infant to nurse. I suspect that your memory of the tragedy will be short-lived and fade with time.

For Mary Ann's parents there will be ongoing hopes that will never be met. There will be no first birthday, first day of kindergarten, no prom, no graduation, no college, no giving away of the bride and countless other unfulfilled dreams.

I have been a physician for 45 years. This is the worst case of negligence I have seen. Not knowing the baby was breech does not meet any standard of care. Your arrogance and/or ignorance by not listening to the mother to call 911 resulted in the death of an innocent and defenseless infant.

All of your unbelievable mistakes will be enumerated as we proceed filing formal complaints. You should never be allowed to deliver another infant.

Yesterday, Mary Ann's parents returned to Denver with a small coffin.

Paul N. Tschetter, MD

Complaint to the Washington State Health Department

On February 2, 2006, I filed a complaint about Pamela Golliet's negligent practice of medicine resulting in the death of our granddaughter with the Washington State Health Department. The thrust of the complaint was as follows:

- Ms. Golliet did a home delivery for our son and daughter-in-law on January 18, 2006. The baby was born breech and was severely compromised at birth. The infant did not get to Providence St. Peter Hospital ER for about 25–40 minutes where she was resuscitated and put on life support. She then was transported to Tacoma General Hospital. The second EEG showed no brain activity and life support was discontinued on January 21, 2006.
- Failure to diagnose the baby was breech: If it was known that the baby was breech, a C-Section would have been done, and the baby would have been fine. The baby was 40 weeks (term) and weighed 8 lbs. Just before delivery, Ms. Golliet still thought the baby was head down and commented that she "could feel the baby's hair." She was feeling the infant's buttock. After the

body was delivered, she couldn't deliver the head for five minutes. Imagine the horrible scene.
- *Prolonged second-stage labor.* An estimated 2nd Stage of 6–8 hours should have been an indication there was a problem. Mother should have been taken to the hospital. Since the only pelvic exam that was done was at the onset of labor, there was no way to know when full dilatation—the start of 2nd Stage—occurred.
- *Inadequate emergency plan.* Calling 911 would not be an inappropriate plan. In an emergency, time is a large factor. The baby did not get to the ER in a timely manner and irreversible brain damage had occurred. Taking mother to the hospital early on as she requested would have been a good emergency plan.
- *Inadequate resuscitation plan.* With proper medical equipment, Ms. Golliet should have been able to intubate the baby at once and support respiration. The only equipment she had was a rubber bulb syringe and an oxygen tank.
- *Attempting a vaginal birth after C-Section (VBAC) at home.* VBACs are high risk, and 30% require a C-Section. If you are doing a VBAC, immediate C-Section capability must be available. This capability is only available in a hospital.
- *Inadequate training.* It is doubtful that Ms. Golliet is trained to deliver a breech presentation or do a VBAC. We have since learned that Ms. Golliet was licensed in February 2005! She had told the parents

that she had done many deliveries including VBACs. She may have been present at deliveries, but certainly in an 11-month time she had not done a large number of deliveries. We doubt she has ever delivered a breech baby.
- *Failure to use a backup obstetrician.* We do not know if a midwife is required to have backup or not in Washington State. I can't imagine that one is not required.
- *Failure to get an ultrasound.* Ms. Golliet was concerned about the baby's position several weeks before the due date and recommended that mother see a chiropractor. Mother saw Jeanine Wolf-Richter who used the "Webster Technique" to "relax the pelvic ligaments so the baby could get in the right position." It was obvious and this confirms that Ms. Golliet was concerned about position.
- Neither Ms. Golliet nor the chiropractor performed an ultrasound to check the baby's position.
- *Failure to heed mother's cry for help.* "Call 911 and take me to the hospital!" At that point, if mother had gone to the hospital, an ultrasound would have been done, followed by a C-Section and the baby's life would have been saved.
- *Informed consent.* I have not seen the document, but I doubt the high risk of a VBAC was clearly presented. The parents were told by Golliet that she had "successfully done 10–12 VBACs." I doubt Ms. Golliet could document the accuracy of this representation.

- As we learn more about this tragic event, there may be more complaints.
- We respectfully request an investigation. Pending the results of said investigation, we urge you to immediately revoke Golliet's license before she kills another baby.
- On or about February 22, 2006, I spoke with Sandy Pridaux. Ms. Pridaux was with the Washington Department of Health. I told her that when the 2nd Stage labor started is unknown because Golliet only performed a single pelvic exam at the onset of labor. Ms. Pridaux acknowledged that a single pelvic exam during a 24-hour labor is totally inadequate.
- During labor, mother repeatedly requested for Golliet to perform pelvic exams but Golliet failed to do so. Mother repeatedly requested to be examined.
- Golliet's answer to my wife Renee's question, "Are you sure the head is down?" was wrong.
- Ms. Golliet has no credibility. At best, Golliet misrepresented her background and at worst she lied when she told these parents she had been doing deliveries for 20 years.
- Golliet was negligent in not having appropriate equipment to resuscitate the baby. It is doubtful that Golliet had Pediatric Advanced Life Support training (PALS) or even newborn life support training.
- Golliet's changing of her website the day after the baby was delivered is an admission that the representations made on her web-

site regarding her background and experience were false.

The hearing is set, 2008

In February 2008, our son informed me that the Washington State assistant attorney general contacted him. Mary Ann's wrongful death case was now set for hearing August 11–14, 2008.

Both parents would likely be called to testify on the eleventh. The State of Washington was going to pay for their travel and lodging. Sometime in April, depositions were scheduled to take place in Colorado. These depositions were never taken. The State of Washington never explained to the parents why they were not given an opportunity to testify how Golliet had killed their baby.

The experts

Gail Hart, LDEM

Gail Hart, LDEM (licensed direct entry midwife), was selected to give her opinions regarding the care of mother and Mary Ann. Hart had been a certified practical midwife since 1976 and an LDEM since 1994. She was now semiretired and no longer maintained her license, but still kept active with a small community practice. Hart opined that Golliet's prenatal care was appropriate. Hart identified hypertension as a risk factor. Despite the fact that Golliet failed to monitor mother's hypertension, by taking appropriate blood pressure readings during labor, Hart opined that mother's hypertension was properly monitored.

Hart offered the following additional observations and opinions:

- Labor continued as anticipated until the surprise breech.
- She speculated that the baby might have turned into the breech position during labor. A surprise breech is known to occur, and even a long-term practicing midwife may misdiagnose a breech.

- During the breech extraction, Golliet performed well within the standard of care and handled the use of CPR and calling emergency personnel.
- It was approximately six minutes from the time the heart rate dropped until the delivery was complete. This time frame is well within the time required to complete a proper breech extraction. Thus a baby in that situation should be just fine after delivery.

Overall, Hart concluded that Golliet's handling of mother and Mary Ann was appropriate and complied with the standard of care of a reasonably competent midwife. Therefore a breach of the standard of care did not cause Mary Ann's death.

In a stunning, unbelievable, and surreal total miscarriage of justice, no one was ever given the opportunity to question Hart regarding her totally unfounded and incompetent opinions. The most basic cross-examination would have forced Hart to admit that her opinions and conclusions were based on the huge assumption that Mary Ann became breech when she turned during labor. An assumption that was totally contradicted by the fact that Golliet sent mother to the chiropractor to turn the baby.

My personal questions/statements of Hart, had I been given the opportunity, were as follows:

- An assumption that would not have been an assumption if Golliet had met the standard of care by having an ultrasound done during prenatal care.
- Ms. Hart, we can agree that we would have 100% certainty that Mary Ann was not breech if an ultrasound had been performed at any time prior to delivery.
- Ms. Hart, we can also agree that Ms. Golliet never performed an ultrasound predelivery despite having knowledge that the baby might be in a breech position.

- How is this not a violation of the duty of care?
- How can you opine that mother's prenatal care was appropriate given Golliet's failure to perform an ultrasound under these circumstances?
- Isn't it a violation of the standard of care to fail or refuse to call 911 after the mother delivering the baby specifically instructs you to call 911?

Charles Petty, MD

Charles Petty, MD, is board-certified in OB-GYN and Internal Medicine. He completed both of his residencies at the University of Washington. He has combined this seemingly disparate training into a career in high-risk pregnancies at Swedish Medical Center, Seattle, Washington, for over forty years.

Dr. Petty's review of the records soundly rebutted Gail Hart's opinions. Thorough review of the records accordingly led him to the opposite and sound conclusion: Golliet did not meet the standard of care of a reasonable and prudent licensed midwife in the State of Washington in her care of mother and Mary Ann. Ms. Golliet's actions were unprofessional and negligent, incompetent, and therefore constituted malpractice. Golliet's actions were the direct cause of the death of Mary Ann, a newborn infant.

Specially, Pamela Golliet did not meet the standard of care of a reasonable and prudent midwife in the state of Washington for the following reasons:

1. She failed to recognize the breech position of the fetus before and during labor. The failure to diagnose the breech presentation was the proximate cause of the difficult delivery and subsequent death of this newborn. The infant was well into the birth canal on 12/28/05. It is probable

that the infant was breech at that time. It would be "very unlikely" the fetus could spontaneously turn from head down to breech. The exam done in early labor shows a 7 cm dilatation and a 1+ station. Ms. Golliet should have been able to feel the landmarks of the fetal head with certainty. The fact that she did not make the diagnosis of breech presentation showed a lack of ability and/or experience. This is below the standard of care. (She had only had her license for 11 months.)

2. Her delivery of this breech infant was done in a manner that caused great harm to the newborn. Specifically, the manner or delivery caused prolonged oxygen deprivation which resulted in hypoxic ischemic encephalopathy, multiple organ failure and death. Had Ms. Golliet recognized when the fetal buttocks were visible at the opening of the vagina, she could have had mother stop pushing and called 911. This would have allowed mother time to get to the hospital in time for an emergency C-section which would have saved Mary Ann's life. Even the father realized what he saw was not his daughter's head. After about 25 minutes, Ms. Golliet asked him if he wanted to feel the baby's head and he told her, "That is not a head." Ms. Golliet disagreed with him. Dr. Petty comments that Ms. Golliet postulated even now that the head was down for most of the labor and somehow turned to breech. "This simply is not possible," Dr. Hart opined. Ms. Golliet does not recall mother asking for another ultrasound. Ms. Golliet states she felt confident in her palpation skills for the baby's position. Dr. Petty further comments that Ms. Golliet did not realize then, nor does she acknowledge now, that she was badly mistaken during the entire labor about

the fetus' position. She seemed unaware that she could learn something from this tragedy.

3. Golliet's delivery of this breech infant was done in such a manner that great harm was done to the newborn. Delivery caused prolonged oxygen deprivation which resulted in hypoxic ischemic encephalopathy, multiple organ failure and death. The parents said that Ms. Golliet panicked with the realization that she had a breech on her hands. Instead of remaining calm and assisting mother in a gentle delivery, she had mother push harder and she reached into the vagina and pulled on the baby in an ill-advised attempt to hasten the delivery.

4. Golliet failed to follow her own guidelines and the accepted standard of care in regard to hypertension during labor, which required the transfer of mother to the hospital for management and delivery. All of the recorded BPs were over 140/90. The highest was 152/104. All of the BPs were high enough to require immediate transfer to the hospital. She [Golliet] apparently solved the problem by not taking any more blood pressures. Ms. Golliet did not meet the standard of care when she failed to consult with a physician and transfer to the hospital for delivery. This failure put both the mother and the fetus at increased risk. For the mother, the risk includes seizures and stroke; and, for the fetus decreased amniotic fluid, fetal heart abnormalities, and placental abruption which in fact did occur.

5. A direct consequence of mother's hypertension during labor was placental abruption, which further compromised the newborn; appropriate transfer would have avoided this complication.

6. Ms. Golliet failed to provide antibiotics to mother during labor. Mother was known to be Group B streptococcus positive and antibiotics are indicated for prevention of newborn Group B streptococcus disease.
7. Ms. Golliet billed DSHS [an insurance company] for a home delivery. Since mother had a previous Cesarean delivery, she was not eligible for DSHS coverage for a home delivery. The reason a home delivery after C-Section is not covered is because the risk of complications is too high.

Another complaint against Golliet

At some point, we were told that the doctors on the Providence St. Peter's Quality Control Committee also filed a complaint against Golliet. However, because we were never provided a copy of the complaint, we are uncertain whether it was filed and what the allegations were against Golliet.

The secret emails

At some point in time, we learned that multiple emails were exchanged between the Washington State Health Department and Golliet's attorney. We also learned that the Washington State attorney general's office was copied on these emails. The emails apparently were settlement discussions between Golliet, her attorney, the Department of Health, and the attorney general's office. However, we don't know for certain because the copies of the emails that we received were completely redacted. The only information that was not redacted was who sent and received the emails and the date the emails were sent. No one ever offered an explanation or provided justification as to why the contents of the emails were redacted. No explanation was provided as to why Mary Ann's parents (the victims of Golliet's criminal conduct) were not included or allowed to weigh in on these discussions.

The surprise settlement

The August 2008 hearing never took place! Golliet's attorney and the Washington State Health Department reached a stipulated settlement of the matter (a plea bargain). We had absolutely zero input or knowledge of the settlement. We only learned of the settlement from the doula who attended the delivery.

After learning of the settlement, our son and daughter-in-law left a voicemail for the attorney at the attorney general's (AG) office. The attorney eventually responded on July 15, 2008, and said that he would talk to them after he returned from his long-planned vacation. He had not called sooner due to his very busy litigation schedule. Because the stipulated settlement was signed by Golliet on June 20, 2008, we thought regardless of his schedule, certainly he could have found time to call during the intervening twenty-five-day period. The fact that the stipulated settlement was probably reached much earlier, as early as May, made the total lack of communication even worse. The AG's callous failure to timely communicate with mother and father, or to include them in the settlement process, was clear evidence of their indifference. The Washington State AG's office appeared to care less that Golliet had killed Mary Ann. Given my outrage over the situation, I attempted to talk to the AG attorney, but he would never take my call.

STIPULATIONS, FINDINGS OF FACT, AND CONCLUSIONS OF LAW

Procedural Stipulations:

- On August 6, 2007, the Washington State Department of Health (the State) issued a Statement of Charges against the Respondent, Pamela Golliet.
- The State alleges that Respondent violated RCW 18.130.180(4) ("Incompetence, negligence, or malpractice which results in injury to a patient or which creates an unreasonable risk that a patient may be harmed. The use of a nontraditional treatment by itself shall not constitute unprofessional conduct, provided that it does not result in injury to a patient or create an unreasonable risk that a patient may be harmed.")
- The State is prepared to proceed to a hearing on the allegations.
- If the allegations are proven, the Secretary of Health has the power to impose sanctions.
- Respondent has the right to defend against the allegations.

The Finding of Fact—Respondent and the Program stipulate to the following facts:

- On February 1, 2005 The Respondent was issued credentials to practice as a midwife.
- Between November, 2005 and January, 2006 she provided midwifery services to Patients A and B.
- On January 17 and 18, 2006 the Respondent facilitated the home delivery of Patient B.
- During the delivery The Respondent failed to diagnose that Patient B presented in a breech position, which placed Patients A and B at risk of harm.
- During the delivery, Respondent failed to properly respond to Patient A's elevated blood pressure, which caused risk of patient harm.

Conclusions of Law—Respondent and the State agree to the entry of the following Conclusion of Law:

- Respondent has committed unprofessional conduct in violation of RCW 18.130180(4).
- The above violation provides grounds for imposing sanctions under RCW 18.130.160.

Agreed Order:

- Respondent's credential to practice as a midwife in the state of Washington shall be placed on Probation for at least 36 months. During this time the Respondent shall follow all of the following terms and conditions.
- Respondent shall present both portions of her credentials to the State to be stamped

"probation"…and all subsequent credentials received during this Agreed Order are stamped "probation."
- Respondent is permanently restricted from attending Vaginal Birth After C-Section (VBACs) in home birth settings.
- Respondent is permanently restricted from attending known breech deliveries in home birth settings.
- Respondent must submit a written protocol for attending and managing deliveries for mothers with a history of toxemia and/or preeclampsia.
- Respondent must modify all informed consent documents…so that they identify the restrictions to her practice imposed by the Agreed Order.
- Respondent must submit annual audits by the Department of Health during the probationary period.
- Respondent shall pay a fine of $3,000.
- Respondent shall obey all federal, state and local laws and all administrative rules governing the practice of the profession in Washington.
- If the Respondent violates any provision… the Secretary may take further action against the Respondent's credentials.

Failure to Comply:

- Failure to comply may result in suspension of the credential after a show cause hearing.
- The Secretary may hold a hearing to require the Respondent to show cause why the credential should not be suspended.

- The Secretary may bring additional charges of unprofessional conduct.

Unbelievably and to our great dismay, the findings of fact, conclusions of law and order failed to mention that Mary Ann (patient B) had died due to Golliet's gross negligence! The whole process and result were a sham in our eyes. It also failed to address the many other allegations of malpractice raised in my original complaint.

The unanswered questions

Over a year later, and after discovering more information as to what had actually transpired, we had many unanswered additional questions. These questions were addressed to the Health Systems Quality Assurance, Washington State Department of Health. The most critical questions were as follows:

1. Why was this case settled in secret and without any input or participation from the victim and the complainant?
2. How can a settlement be reached when only Golliet and her lawyer are present? Why was our attorney not allowed to participate in the settlement process and represent Mary Ann and her parents' interests? How can the State of Washington sign off on a document that states "The parties agree to resolve this matter by means of this Agreed Order" when we or our representatives were not part of the process in any way?
3. Why were we not notified of the decision to settle this case? Why were we not notified when the settlement was reached? I filed the complaint and should have been informed of the decision. Mary Ann's parents only learned of the settlement because the doula called them. They should have officially been told this by the assistant attorney general.
4. Why did the stipulated settlement pleading fail to state both that Mary Ann died and that her death was the direct result of Pamela Golliet's gross negligence? The failure to mention the fact that Mary Ann died is an unacceptable miscarriage

of justice. Why? Because the settlement specifically does state that Golliet committed unprofessional conduct in violation of Washington State law. How can the State agree to a settlement that states a midwife committed negligence but fails to mention the devastating consequences of that negligence? If we had been allowed to be involved as we should have, we would have never agreed to anything less than an unequivocal statement that Golliet killed Mary Ann and that she is permanently barred from delivering babies.

All these questions remain unanswered to this day. While initially appearing sympathetic and determined to hold Golliet accountable, those involved for Washington State completely failed to understand our anger and complete frustration over the result. In our view, Washington State got steamrolled by Golliet's noted attorney into a fast and easy settlement without any input from us. While it was fast and easy for Washington State and Golliet, the settlement utterly failed to recognize that Mary Ann had died.

As a pediatrician for forty-nine years, I have dealt with the deaths of too many children. The death of a child is the most difficult death a family can experience. The fact that Golliet received only a slap on the wrist completely insulted Mary Ann's parents and our family. It deepened our pain, making it even more difficult to recover from this tragedy. Over the years, I have testified as an expert witness and reviewed many cases of malpractice. None were even close to the flagrant negligence Golliet exhibited. The State of Washington and all those involved did not give Mary Ann or us any justice. Golliet should not have been allowed to continue to deliver babies.

Epilogue

We filed a complaint against Golliet to prevent her from doing any more deliveries and thus harming other families. Because Washington State did not suspend her license as a result of our complaint, we did not accomplish this goal and assumed Golliet would still be allowed to deliver babies.

However, when I checked again a few years ago, I stumbled across another complaint filed against Golliet in 2011. Many of the facts set forth in the 2011 complaint were similar to how Golliet had botched Mary Ann's birth. In particular, Golliet failed to transport the mother to the hospital when midwife standards dictated that she should due to complications during labor. Similar to Mary Ann's birth, Golliet also failed to monitor key vital signs of the mother during labor. In addition, like Mary Ann's birth, Golliet failed to address streptococcus B. Additional allegations (that differed from Mary Ann's birth) were that Golliet failed to conduct required newborn screening tests and failed to refer the mother to a pediatrician after birth due to the baby's weight loss.

While the publicly available documents in the 2011 complaint do not indicate whether mother or baby died (we presume they did not for this reason), Golliet's wanton and reckless actions during Mary Ann's birth were much worse in our opinion. However, Golliet received a much stiffer punishment as a result of the 2011 complaint: the Washington State Health Department suspended Golliet's midwife license for a period of three (3) years in 2012. This case only reinforced the total miscarriage of justice in Mary Ann's case because Golliet was only placed on probation for three years, when her actions clearly resulted in Mary Ann's death.

Tragedy

The dictionary defines a *tragedy* as "an event causing great suffering, destruction, and distress, such as a serious accident, crime, or natural catastrophe." While Mary Ann's death caused great suffering and distress, I recently heard a better definition of tragedy in a Catholic Homily:

"An event that should have never happened."

Mary Ann's death should never have happened.

MARY ANN
PAUL N. TSCHETTER
JUNE 11, 2007

Your life
So short

You left us
before we knew you

I held you in my arms
As the last flicker of your life
Ebbed silently away

This brief moment
In time
Will become a lifetime
Memory

As your soul commits
Into the hands of God

EPILOGUE

In John Steinbeck's book, *Travels with Charley in Search of America*, he and his dog travel throughout the United States. During their excursion they met many fascinating people and rarely an unsavory character. Steinbeck always kept a good supply of coffee and whiskey while traveling. His conclusion was that life is a journey and not a destination.

My life journey has had much joy and some sadness. Over the years I learned some lessons I want to share.

- Leave this world a better place than you found it.
- Never take more than you give.
- Make all contacts with others a positive experience.

Have a wonderful journey and I hope you enjoyed my book.

ABOUT THE AUTHOR

Dr. Tschetter was raised and attended public schools in Denver, Colorado. He received an academic scholarship to Dartmouth College, where he graduated magna cum laude. He was elected to Phi Beta Kappa his junior year.

Dr. Tschetter continued his education and attended Dartmouth Medical School and the Colorado University School of Medicine, graduating Alpha Omega Alpha Honor Society. He completed his internship and residency at Colorado General Hospital, Denver. He practiced pediatric medicine in the South Metro Denver community for forty-nine years.

During his career, Dr. Tschetter served as president of the medical staff and was on the board of directors at Children's Hospital Colorado. Teaching medical students, interns, and residents was a passion. He was named a career teaching scholar and rose to the rank of clinical professor of pediatrics emeritus. He received many awards, including the Outstanding Service Award and the James E. Strain, MD, Award, honoring pediatricians who exemplify the ideals of the American Academy of Pediatrics and its advocacy for child health.

Dr. Tschetter served on the board of directors for Brent's Place for fifteen years. Brent's Place provides housing for families whose children are undergoing a bone marrow transplant or chemotherapy.

Dr. Tschetter and his wife, Renee, live in Greenwood Village, Colorado. They have seven children, nineteen grandchildren, and four great-grandchildren.